# SENSUAL
# FOR LIFE

# SENSUAL FOR LIFE

## THE NATURAL WAY to MAINTAIN SEXUAL VITALITY

GEORGE L. REDMON, PH.D., N.D.

TWIN STREAMS
Kensington Publishing Corp.
http://www.kensingtonbooks.com

This book presents information based upon the research and personal experiences of the author. It is not intended to be a substitute for a professional consultation with a physician or other healthcare provider. Neither the publisher nor the author can be held responsible for any adverse effects or consequences resulting from the use of any of the information in this book. They also cannot be held responsible for any errors or omissions in the book. If you have a condition that requires medical advice, the publisher and author urge you to consult a competent healthcare professional.

TWIN STREAMS BOOKS are published by

Kensington Publishing Corp.
850 Third Avenue
New York, NY 10022

Figure 1.1 on p. 10 and Figure 1.3 on p. 18 are from *Anatomy and Physiology* by Eva Lurie Weinreb, copyright © 1984 by Addison-Wesley Publishing. They are used by permission of Addison-Wesley Publishing.

Figure 1.2 on p. 12 is from *Textbook of Anatomy and Physiology,* 8th Edition, by Catherine Parker Anthony and Nora Jane Kolthoff, copyright © 1971 by C.V. Mosby Co. It is used by permission of C.V. Mosby Co.

Figure 2.1, A Position for Genital Play, on p. 24 is from *Heterosexuality* by William Masters, Virginia Johnson, and Robert Kolodny, copyright © 1994 by William H. Masters, Virginia E. Johnson, and Robert C. Kolodny. Reprinted by permission of HarperCollins Publishers, Inc.

Figure 2.2 on p. 28 is from *You and Your Hormone Glands* by R.C. Khurana, copyright © 1978 by Obesity and Diabetes Books Publishing. It is used by permission of Obesity and Diabetes Books Publishing.

Figure III.1 on p. 71 and Figure 7.1 on p. 79 are from *Reversing Impotence Forever!* by David F. Mobley and Steven K. Wilson, copyright © 1995 by Swan Publishing. They are used by permission of Swan Publishing.

Figure 7.2 on p. 80 is from *American Sex Machines* by Hoag Levins. Copyright © 1996. Used by permission of Adams Media Corporation. All rights reserved.

Figure 9.1 on p. 105 is from *Natural Hormone Replacement* by Jonathan V. Wright and John Morgenthaler, copyright © 1997 by Smart Publications. It is used by permission of Smart Publications (800-976-2783).

All Kensington titles, imprints, and distributed lines are available at special quantity discounts for bulk purchases for sales promotion, premiums, fund-raising, educational or institutional use.

Special book excerpts or customized printings can also be created to fit specific needs. For details, write or phone the office of the Kensington Special Sales Manager: Kensington Publishing Corp., 850 Third Avenue, New York, NY 10022. Attn: Special Sales Department. Phone: 1-800-221-2647.

Twin Streams and the TS logo Reg. U.S. Pat. & TM Off.

ISBN 0-7582-0138-9

First Trade Printing: March 2003
10 9 8 7 6 5 4 3 2 1

Printed in the United States of America

*This book is dedicated to my father, George Redmon Jr. Thank you for your guidance and undying support and for being the beacon of light that has and still inspires me. I will love you forever!*

# Contents

# Acknowledgments

I will be forever indebted to Mr. Eric Dettrey and his secretarial support staff for their fine efforts and dedication toward the completion of this book.

I would like to give a special thanks to Mrs. Lorri Fioravanti for her individual and exceptional editorial and copy work, without which this project would have been severely compromised. Thank you, Lorri.

As a researcher, I would like to give thanks to the past and present investigators, scientists, and healthcare professionals whose diligence and devotion to the preservation of human life motivate me toward that same cause. I am also sincerely grateful to my editor, Mrs. Elaine Will Sparber of Kensington Publishing, and her colleagues for providing the platform for this topic's review and study.

This author owes a sincere debt of gratitude to my wife, Brenda, and my son, George Jr., for their undying support. Lastly, I would like to acknowledge the following individuals who gave emotional and intellectual support that contributed greatly to the completion of this project: Dr. Suzette T. Avetian, D.O., Mercy Medical Center, Upper Darby, Pennsylvania; Ms. Andrea Foster, Director, The Holistic Resource and Referral Network of Houston, Texas; Dr. Barry Persky, Ph.D., Long Island University, Department of Education, Brooklyn, New York; Dr. Pamela Peters, Ph.D., Director and Founder, The Center for Stress Pain and Wellness Management, Wilmington, Delaware; and Dr. Marcia B. Steinhauer, Ph.D., Department of Health and Human Services, Walden University, Minneapolis, Minnesota.

# Preface

*Many people believe that the late 1960's was a complete understanding of our sexuality, but in fact, the extent of sexual ignorance remains staggering. Lack of knowledge about sex, what I call sexual illiteracy, is an important cause of adult sexual problems.*

Domeena Renshaw, M.D.
Director, Loyola Sex Therapy Clinic

*What I see now is sex without intimacy, sex without pleasure: people trapped in destructive, repetitive habits, doing things they don't want to do, uncertain and afraid to try things they'd like to do—men needing to know more about the sexuality of women, women needing to know about the sexuality of men.*

Debora Phillips, Ph.D.
Associate Clinical Professor,
Temple Medical School

*We now understand that to a great extent the body operates on a "use it or lose it" principle. That is true of heart, mind and muscles. That means that there are ways to make sure you will be as sharp, vital, and alive in thirty years as you are right now!*

Stuart Berger, M.D.
*Forever Young* (William Morrow, 1989)

*Sexual function is one of the last functions to decline with age. Men and women can live sexually fulfilled lives well into their nineties and beyond. All you need are a few guidelines to help keep the fires going.*

Helen S. Kaplan, M.D., Ph.D.
Director, Human Sexuality,
Cornell Medical Center

*For it is possible to continue an active sex life indefinitely.*

Ruth Westheimer, Ph.D.
Host, *Sexually Speaking*
(nationally syndicated radio show)

When you read the above comments by prominent sexual health professionals, you can see that from a biological standpoint, you have the capability to maintain your sexual potency, virility, stamina, drive, and overall sexual health forever! The comments also imply that the rising incidence of sexual dysfunction in America today is at least in part directly related to misinformation and individual lifestyle choices. They also suggest that you, the individual, will throughout your lifetime have the most impact on the restoration, maintenance, and management of the involutional sexual changes you will experience.

As a naturopathic doctor, I am often asked by my male clients (who fall into all age groups) if there is something natural they can take over the course of a few days or hours to help them avoid embarrassing themselves with their lovers. My female clients often ask about products that will increase their interest so that they can perform on a level playing field. One of the more difficult things to get clients to understand is that the manifestation of a metabolic breakdown in many cases is the result of long-term neglect, not listening to the daily signals that the body gives, and more important, treating the symptoms rather than the root causes of problems.

This point really strikes at the heart of the above quotes from the experts in the field of human sexuality. It is the purpose of this book: to give you the opportunity to explore many of the established and new natural alternatives that are available to help you restore, heighten, and maintain your sexual vitality for life.

The overall goal of this book is to help you establish a life-long preventive plan that will keep you sexually active and vibrant. *Sensual for*

*Life* is a book that focuses on sexual health, not sexual dysfunction. Each and every one of us has the biological capability of having and enjoying sexual abilities until the day we die.

Sexual health is maintained by focusing one's efforts on remaining both physically and mentally healthy. One without the other will spell disaster, and will increase the probability that you will never reach or experience your full sexual potential. Our sexual encounters are what connect us to the universe we inhabit, and to the individuals we love. Our sexual ability and contact are what ensure that we remain youthful, motivated, and in many cases healthy, emotionally as well as physically.

According to Henry Bieler, M.D., author of *Dr. Bieler's Natural Way to Sexual Health* (Charles Publishing, 1972) and one of the country's early medical doctors who pioneered the use of alternative medicine and natural remedies, it is important that we understand the invariable changes that occur at the various stages of life. Theresa L. Crenshaw, M.D., a well-known sexual health therapist, identifies these changes in our sexual self as "sexual stages." The key here is realizing that some change in your sexual capabilities and overall sexual health may occur, but that sexual dysfunction itself is not inevitable, nor should it be expected.

As expressed by world-renowned experts and pioneers in the study of human sexuality Bernard D. Starr, Ph.D., and Marcella Bakur Weiner, Ed.D., authors of *The Star-Weiner Report on Sex and Sexuality in the Mature Years* (Stein and Day Publishers, 1981), to develop your sexual potential, you need to overcome the belief that sex is purely a natural function. These researchers maintain that it is a mistake to overestimate the romance of sex and think that working on sexual technique is mechanical or artificial. According to Dr. Starr and Dr. Weiner:

> The possession of a powerful sex drive or capacity for pleasure do not guarantee that your early experience and training will teach you how best to use your "biological equipment." There is reason to consciously develop "new modes" of sexual behavior and response. With knowledge, awareness and a commitment to change everyone can reach a heightened level of sexuality and experience sex forever.

*Sensual for Life* will show you how to negate or slow down the biological changes that occur as you move through your sexual stages. These invariable changes, which I call the invisible hand of nature, although biologically preset, can in many cases be controlled, or slowed down, without surgery or the use of dangerous drugs, which in the end can compromise your overall health and will in all probability prevent you from realizing, reaching, or enjoying your full sexual potential.

As stated by Helen S. Kaplan, M.D., Ph.D., director of Human Sexuality at Cornell Medical Center and considered a world-renowned expert in the aspects of human sexuality, "Sexual function is one of the last functions to decline with age."

So in reality, and from a purely biological standpoint, based on scientific fact, you are capable in the absence of any congenital defects of having sex every day of your life. And I mean sex that is full of excitement, adventure, diversity, and imagination, coupled with emotional fulfillment, orgasmic zest, and zeal.

All you need is a plan. *Sensual for Life* will help you formulate a plan of action. While the protocols are intended to help with maintaining sexual health, many of them can be used to help restore lost libido, as well as combat other sexual disorders.

You will find that your best weapon against disturbances of your sexual health is you! Many of your friends, relatives, and coworkers will invariably encounter setbacks in realizing their sexual potential and will resort to dangerous drugs or surgery. You, on the other hand, by making a few changes and adhering to the recommendations outlined in this book, can watch them from the sidelines in tip-top shape and health, physically, mentally, and emotionally. More important, you will enhance your ability to have and enjoy great sex, in each and every encounter, for the rest of your life!

# Introduction

Estimates indicate that 10 to 20 million American men and women suffer from some sort of sexual dysfunction. It is a known fact that we are living longer, and population studies show that within the next several decades, there will be an explosion in the number of adults over the age of 60. This is in great contrast to our life expectancy several decades ago. In fact, present-day antiaging researchers such as Robert Goldman, M.D., D.O., Ph.D., founder and chairman of the American Academy of Anti-Aging Medicine and coauthor of *Stopping the Clock* (Keats Publishing, 1996), maintain that individuals born today can expect to live well into their seventies, and that if current life expectancy trends continue, the average life span for males may reach 100.

These same possibilities exist for women today as current projections suggest that in the next ten years alone, more than 20 million American women will go through menopause. Laura E. Corio, M.D., a board-certified physician specializing in obstetrics and gynecology at the Mount Sinai Medical Center in New York City and author of *The Change Before the Change* (Bantam Books, 2000), makes note of the fact that as of the year 2000, a total of 50 million American women—one-third of the female population—are of perimenopausal or menopausal age.

As a point of reference here, perimenopause is the transitional stage between the reproductive years and menopause. Although the average age of menopause is 51, perimenopause usually begins in the forties and can last for two to eight years or longer.

What do numbers have to do with sex? Everything! A case in point:

As recently as in 1900, according to Frank Kendig and Richard Hutton, authors of *Life Spans, or How Long Things Last* (Henry Holt and Company, 1979), the average life span of men was only 46.3 years. These authors made note of the fact that peak male sexuality, the "prime time stuff," happened between the ages of 14 and 15, when men matured. Their findings show that for thousands of years men's sexuality peaked at 14 or 15 then sexual activity continued until they died at around 45.

As we have just learned, current data show that men have an additional 30 years of sexual capability owing to the increase in their life expectancy. However, a survey that appeared in the *Journal of the American Medical Association* on February 10, 1999, found that sexual dysfunction was actually more prevalent in women. Of the 1,749 women and the 1,410 men between the ages of 18 and 59 who responded, 43 percent of the women reported some form of sexual dysfunction as compared to 31 percent of the men.

When you read data like this, you wonder how much of the problems reported by the respondents can be directly related to their past and present lifestyle choices. In addition, two key questions come to mind:

1. Are we capable of maintaining our sexual health beyond the new median age range of 37.5 to 46.3 years without the use of drugs or surgery?
2. Is aging itself a direct cause of what many people believe to be inevitable problems in maintaining sexual health?

The answer to question number one is a rousing yes! And the answer to question number two is an astounding no!

As expressed by Carlton Fredericks, Ph.D., a pioneer in the medical application of nutrition and supplements; although aging is linked to a number of degenerative diseases, it is not necessarily a cause. In other words, loss of sexual ability may not be directly related to aging. In fact, Deepak Chopra, M.D., one of the world's foremost and most well-known medical professionals, states:

> Over time, various age changes, as gerontologists call them, exert massive influence. But at any given moment, aging accounts for only 1 percent per year of the total change taking

place inside your body. In other words, 99 percent of the energy and intelligence that you are composed of is untouched by the aging process.

One of the major obstacles that may prevent us from realizing our full sexual potential is our own obstinacy. In our society, historically, we suppress the need to know about sexuality, early and often, right on up through adulthood. This attitude extends into our middle years and then into our senior years. Our true sexual self throughout much of our life remains a deep dark secret, hidden and never touched or talked about. However, to fully enjoy our sexual capabilities, we need to know and understand the basic rudiments not only of our own sexual anatomy and physiology, but also of those of our partner. It also is of vital importance that we explore our own erotic zones, to fully understand how we respond to sexual stimuli.

The aim of this book is to help you establish a plan of action that will keep you sexually healthy and vibrant not only in the years before you reach the new median age range, but well beyond those years as well.

# PART I

# UNDERSTANDING
# HUMAN SEXUALITY

*Accurate sex education can prevent the needless anxiety and guilt that often surround healthy, normal adult sexuality. In my experience, an overwhelming number of adult sexual problems are rooted in sexual unawareness and early sexual misinformation, which often lead to deep-seated sexual inhibitions.*

Domeena Renshaw, M.D.
*Director, Loyola Sex Therapy Clinic*

Before we begin this fantastic voyage into the dynamic, energy-filled, and—yes—erotic nature of human sexuality, let's explore the central theme of Part I. It is not the author's intent to suggest that you as an adult female or male haven't the slightest idea about your own sexuality. My goal here is to increase your "sexual literacy," as noted sex therapist Dr. Ruth Westheimer calls it, and your knowledge of how your sex organs work biologically.

You have within you a force that could be compared to the hard drive of the most efficient and powerful computer known to humankind. While it may be difficult to comprehend, essentially you transfer and transform vital nutrients and substances to energy that assists nature in perpetuating and maintaining life. To ensure that this process repeats itself, nature has built within you a permanent "sexual blueprint." This blueprint is activated when you are sexually aroused or stimulated. So elaborate is this system that under the right conditions, it will work for you during the entire span of your lifetime. Yes, that is worth repeating: *It will work for you during the entire span of your lifetime!* The key words here are *under the right conditions*. In Part I, therefore, we shall review:

- The basic anatomy and physiology of both the male and the female sexual systems.
- The internal glands that produce the sex hormones that fuel your sexual communication system and your sexual desire and that

have a strong influence on your sexual appetite. They form what we will refer to as the biological basis of your sexual desire.

- The myth of aging and its effect on the sex drive, emotions, and desire. Contrary to popular belief, in the absence of any congenital defects your sexual potential extends through your life span.

The goal of Part I as stated is to increase your "sexual literacy" and your knowledge of how your sex organs work and of the nature of sensuality. This is because a professional-based belief is that the key to cultivating, preserving, maintaining, and managing your life-long sexual health starts here with you and your knowledge of how your sexual systems operate.

No problem, including a sexual one, can be resolved without first knowing the rudiments and the sequence of events that facilitate proper functioning in the first place. This is the point argued by Domeena Renshaw, M.D., director of the Loyola Sex Therapy Clinic in Chicago, on the preceeding page.

For many of us, sexual health is something we take for granted until it begins to falter. Remaining sexually active can become a driving force larger than life itself at times. For many of us, our sexuality simply put defines our existence, our happiness, and what makes us human beings.

It is a professionally based belief that a mechanical view of sexuality will increase your chances of becoming sexually dysfunctional. The more aware you are of the highs and lows of this unique communication system, the better your chances are that you will be able to manage and enjoy your sexual potential through your life span. Understanding your sexuality is your first step toward enjoying it in prime fashion *forever!*

# 1

⚛

# Sexual Anatomy 101

*Basic to the understanding of human sexuality is an accurate knowledge of sexual physiology and functioning—in effect, how the male and female sexual systems work.*

James Leslie McCary, M.D.
*McCary's Human Sexuality*
(Van Nostrand Reinhold, 1978)

The first step in creating an environment that will help you preserve your sexual potential is understanding your body's mechanism of action and reaction. When you look at your heterosexual counterpart, you see that despite the visual physical differences, there exist many similarities in your sexual blueprint and in your sexual response to stimuli. In fact, your external sexual organs actually had the same origins during fetal development. (See Figure 1.1.) The clitoris (a female organ) and the penis (a male organ) start out as identical structures.

Additionally, during sexual arousal, both of you go through several stages before you reach orgasm. As you will see, many of your physical reactions are similar. The stages, as cited by William H. Masters, M.D., and Virginia E. Johnson D.Sc., in *Human Sexual Response* (Little, Brown and Company, 1966), are:

1. *The excitement phase.* This phase develops in response to any form of stimulation.

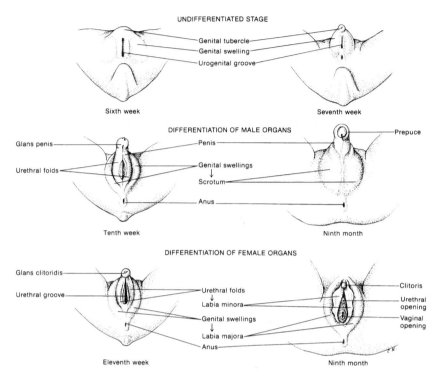

**FIGURE 1.1.** The male and female external genital organs develop from the same structure during the undifferentiated stage of fetal development.

Source: Eva Lurie Weinreb, *Anatomy and Physiology* (Reading, MA: Addison-Wesley Publishing, 1984), p. 776.

2. *The plateau phase.* During this phase of continued sexual stimulation, sexual excitement is intensified.
3. *The orgasmic phase.* During this phase, a state of full sexual arousal is reached and orgasm or ejaculation occurs.
4. *The resolution phase.* At this time, sexual tension resolves and the body returns to its original, unstimulated stage.

During this four-step process from sexual excitement through orgasm, both males and females experience similar physical changes, as cited in Table 1.1.

As you can see from Table 1.1, there are several similarities in func-

## TABLE 1.1.
## BODILY CHANGES DURING SEXUAL AROUSAL

| Female Bodily Changes | Male Bodily Changes |
| --- | --- |
| 1. *Excitement Phase*<br>Vagina becomes wet and moist<br>Vagina starts to enlarge<br>Heart rate and blood pressure<br>increase<br>Nipples become erect, breasts enlarge<br><br>2. *Plateau Phase*<br>Vagina becomes wetter, then subsides,<br>then exudes more fluid as stimula-<br>tion continues<br>Vaginal lips swell and change color<br>Red flushing of skin known as sex flush<br>increases<br>Breathing becomes rapid and shallow<br><br>3. *Orgasmic Phase*<br>Intense contractions of the uterus and<br>rectum occur<br>Heart rate increases<br>Sex flush spreads and intensifies<br><br>4. *Resolution Phase*<br>Clitoris goes back to normal size<br>Heartbeat and respiration return to<br>normal<br>Vaginal lips return to normal size<br>Sex flush subsides<br>State of relaxation begins | 1. *Excitement Phase*<br>Penis begins to enlarge<br>Nipples become erect<br>Heart rate and blood pressure<br>increase<br>Scrotal skin thickens, testes<br>elevate<br><br>2. *Plateau Phase*<br>Penis becomes much firmer,<br>harder, and fuller<br>Testes increase slightly in size<br>Sex flush intensifies<br>Blood pressure rises<br>Breathing becomes rapid and<br>shallow<br><br>3. *Orgasmic Phase*<br>Powerful contractions of pros-<br>tate, rectum, seminal vesicles,<br>and penis occur<br>Heart rate increases<br>Sex flush heightens in intensity<br><br>4. *Resolution Phase*<br>Penis resumes normal soft and<br>limp state<br>Heartbeat and respiration return<br>to normal<br>Testes and scrotum descend<br>Sex flush diminishes<br>State of relaxation begins |

tion, although your physical structures are different. Essentially, your responses to sexual stimuli are the same. It is your sexual apparatus that is different. Let's start by taking a look at the basic anatomical structure of the female sexual system, followed by a review of the male sexual system.

# Female Sexual Anatomy

Mons veneris. Clitoral hood. Clitoral tip. Clitoral glans. Labia majora. Labia minora. Urethra. Vagina. Perineum. Anus. Hymen. How familiar are you with these terms? These terms describe the parts of the female anatomical structure, more commonly known as the female genitalia.

As shown in Figure 1.2, the external section of the female genitals has many different parts. Collectively, these parts are known as the vulva (not to be confused with the vagina). The mound above the pubic area, the mons pubis, or mons veneris, includes the fatty flesh covered by pubic hair. According to Jennifer Berman, M.D., and Laura Berman, Ph.D., codirectors of the Center for Pelvic Medicine at the University of California at Los Angeles, many women find this area to be highly erotic when direct pressure is applied to it. The labia (which is Latin for "lips") is composed of the folds of soft skin that surround the vaginal

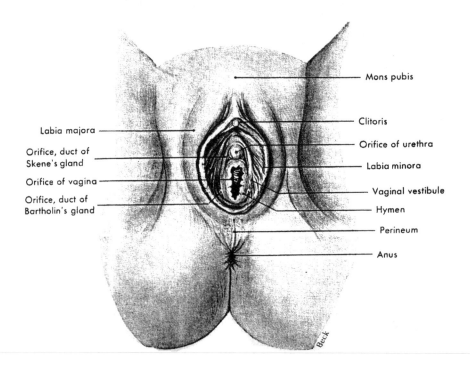

**FIGURE 1.2.** The female genitalia.

**Source:** Catherine Parker Anthony and Nora Jane Kolthoff, *Textbook of Anatomy and Physiology,* 8th Edition (St. Louis, MO: C.V. Mosby Co., 1971), p. 479.

opening. The labia majora are the two larger outer lips, composed of fatty tissue covered with hair. The smaller inner lips, the labia minora, do not grow hair on them. Rather, the labia minora are smooth and moist, and contain a hoard of small blood vessels. During sexual arousal, both of these organs become filled with blood and actually part to allow easier penetration into the vagina. Because of their sensitive nerve endings, the labias are prime target areas for self- and reciprocal stimulation and sexual arousal. The labia minora are highly sensitive.

Along with the above, the labias act much like the locked doors to Fort Knox. They protect the vaginal opening against the harmful contaminants of the outside world, such as molds, dirt, and bacteria. Because of their moist nature, the vaginal walls attract these and other harmful agents.

In addition to the mons pubis and the labias, the female genitalia include the following parts.

## Anus

The anus, as you know, is the site where waste products are expelled. While vaginal intercourse is widely accepted as normal, anal intercourse, for many heterosexual couples, is psycholgically challenging. It is estimated that regardless of the initial psychological barriers, more than half of the adult population would be sexually aroused by anal stimulation. This is due in part to the fact that the anus and genital areas, according to Alfred C. Kinsey, M.D., share some common muscles. Dr. Kinsey and his colleagues at the Kinsey Institute for Research in Sex, Gender, and Reproduction, affiliated with Indiana University, found that when anal stimulation occurred in both females and males, sexual stimulation of the genitals also occurred. In other words, erotic stimulation of the anal area can cause excitement and contraction of the muscles that are involved in sexual arousal of both the male and the female genitalia.

## Breasts

While the breasts are not one of the female external sexual organs, they are highly erotic to many men, according to Peggy Morgan and the editors of *Prevention* magazine in *The Female Body: An Owner's Manual* (Rodale Press, 1996). These authors make note of the fact that like other parts of the body, the breasts contain arteries, veins, and nerve fibers.

The nipples become erect (hard and firm) during the excitement phase of sexual response. The breast, like the male penis, increases in size due to the engorgement of blood as sexual stimulation moves the woman toward the plateau phase. The areola, the darker area surrounding the nipple, also undergoes changes in color and size during sexual arousal.

## G-Spot

The G-spot is located on the upper wall of the vagina and is said to be highly sensitive to sexual manipulation. Sex therapists contend that the G-spot is responsible for what is described by women as ejaculating like a man. Women who first experience this phenomenon become frightened and believe they are urinating. However, researchers say this "female ejaculatory" response is highly pleasurable and is never experienced by many women. Barbara Keesling, Ph.D., author of *Sexual Pleasure* (Hunter House, 1993), says the fluid expelled with a G-spot orgasm is not urine. According to Dr. Keesling, the fluid is thin, much like male ejaculate, but without any sperm. The fluid also is comparable in compositon to prostate fluid.

In Chapter 12, "Holistic Sex Secrets," we will cover the G-spot in more detail, discussing how you or your partner can find and manually manipulate this area. As stated, G-spot orgasms can be highly stimulating and highly energizing.

## Bartholin's Glands

The glands partially responsible for the female secretions are known as the Bartholin's glands. The openings of the two Bartholin's glands are just outside the vagina, in the area sexual-health researchers refer to as the vestibule. This is where the secretions are released. From a purely sexual standpoint, the rapid release of these highly erotic secretions, which happens during heightened sexual arousal, is not only pleasurable to the woman but also highly stimulating to her sexual partner.

The Bartholin's secretions also can be thought of as protectors of the human species. The secretions play an important role in the preservation of sperm cells, as they enter the vagina during sexual intercourse and ejaculation, and help to neutralize its normally acidic environment. This allows the sperm cells to move freely toward their destination, the female egg.

However, for women near their menopausal years, this delicate balance begins to change and the vagina starts to become more alkaline. This can lead to increased susceptibility to yeast, bacterial, and urinary-tract infections. Susceptibility increases due to declining levels of the female hormone estrogen. As pH levels reach 6.0 to 8.0, the acidic nature of the vagina decreases. Vaginal pH this high fosters an environment conducive to the overgrowth of yeast, fungi, and bacteria within the vagina. Healthcare professionals refer to these infections as vaginitis.

The pH scale researchers use runs from 0 to 14. From 0 to 6 is acidic, 7 is neutral, and 8 to 14 is alkaline. A normal pH range for the vagina is 3.5 to 4.5. We will discuss pH and sexuality in more detail in Chapter 9, "Proper Nutrition—Your Best Aphrodisiac," and again in Chapter 11, "Detoxify to Satisfy."

At this point, it is important to know that pH levels too high or too low can derail your sexual potential, not to mention your health.

## Clitoris

The clitoris is one of the most sensitive and erotic organs found on the female body. In fact, the renowned sexual-health investigators Masters and Johnson tell us that the main purpose of the clitoris is to serve both as a receptor and as a transformer of sexual stimuli. These researchers maintain that this organ's only function is to heighten and enhance sexual arousal. Masters and Johnson also note that within the anatomical (external) structure of the human male, no sexual organ exists solely for increasing sexual gratification or pleasure.

Because of the anatomical structure and very small size (just over an inch in length) of the clitoris, many males and females tend to misunderstand the importance of stimulating this part of the female genitals. How important is this action, whether via self-, oral, or manual stimulation? *Extremely important!* In fact, world-renowned sex researcher Dr. Kinsey and his colleagues found that many females never reach maximum arousal without sufficient stimulation of the clitoris. As shown in Figure 1.1, the clitoris is located just above the urethral opening (the tube through which you urinate). Most of the clitoris is covered by soft tissue known as the hood, or prepuce (the clitoral foreskin). Under this hood lies an intricate network of glands that contain erectile tissue called the corpora cavernosa. This highly sensitive tissue, much like the male penis, becomes engorged with blood, causing the clitoris to become erect (hard and stiff). While the clitoris doesn't hang down the way the male penis does, it increases in size and protrudes from its hooded cover when sexually aroused. In fact, sexual-health experts often cite the similarities between the male penis and the female clitoris.

## Perineum

The perineum is located between the vaginal opening and the anus. It is the perineum that medical professionals slightly cut to facilitate easier childbirth. The cut is made right before delivery and repaired immediately afterward.

From a sexual standpoint, the perineum contains nerves that, like the majority of the nerves found within the female as well as the male genitalia, are highly sensitive to the touch. The perineums in both males and females are essentially the same and should be considered prime erotic zones.

## Hymen

The hymen is a thin layer of tissue found near or sometimes partially covering the vaginal opening in younger women. It can be torn during sexual intercourse, exercise, or masturbation, or by the use of tampons.

## Skene's Glands

The Skene's glands, also known as the paraurethral glands, are located within the vagina. They are found near the urethra, alongside the bladder. They open into the Bartholin's glands. The Skene's glands are tiny mucus-producing glands. Located near the G-spot, they produce the fluid that is expelled with a G-spot orgasm.

## Urethra

The urethra, also called the urethral meatus, or urinary opening, is located between the clitoris and the vaginal opening. The urethra is the tube through which the urine flows from the bladder out of the body. Unlike the way both urine and semen pass through the male urethra, only urine passes through the female urethra.

The urethra in women is sometimes mistaken for the clitoris because of their proximity to each other. Sexual-health investigators have found that the urethra is highly sensitive. However, many sexual-health therapists do not recommend engaging in urethral stimulation due to the high possibility of irritation and urinary-tract infection.

## Vagina

The vagina, not to be confused with the vulva, is the opening above the anus and the perineum. During heterosexual intercourse, the male penis is inserted in the vagina. In adolescence, the vagina begins to develop a deep, dark reddish color and to secrete a thick, sticky mucus whose consistency generally remains constant up to menopausal age, which is about 51. This mucus, which is exuded during sexual arousal, is scientifically known as transudation. The wetter the vaginal walls are, the easier is penetration by the male penis and the more fluid, pleasurable, and rhythmic is coitus (sexual intercourse).

# Male Sexual Anatomy

One of the basic differences between the male and the female external genitalia is the visible nature of the male sexual organ. (See Figure 1.3.) This difference begins with the penis.

The penis consists of two parts: the shaft and the glans. The glans is the head of the penis. The opening in the glans is called the meatus. The shaft is covered by a thin layer of skin. Beneath this thin layer of skin, within the shaft, are three cylindrical, spongy bodies of erectile tissue. Two columns of this erectile tissue are known as the corpora cavernosa and run parallel along the length of the penis. The other column, known as the corpus spongiosum, is found at the tip of the penis, and surrounds and protects the urethra. When men are sexually stimulated, it is the corpora cavernosa that become engorged with blood. The erection subsides when the blood leaves these tissues. This is why lifestyle factors such as high cholesterol levels, diabetes, heart disease, and poor circulation to the pelvic area can prevent a man from sustaining an erection long enough to engage in sexual intercourse.

In addition to the corpora cavernosa and corpus spongiosum, the male genitalia include the following parts.

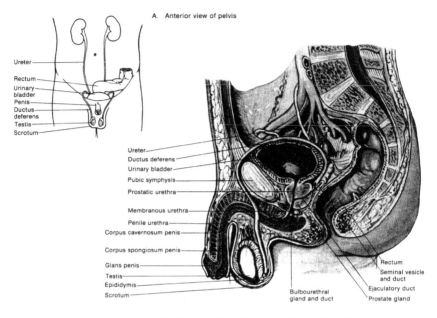

A. Anterior view of pelvis

Ureter
Rectum
Urinary bladder
Penis
Ductus deferens
Testis
Scrotum

Ureter
Ductus deferens
Urinary bladder
Pubic symphysis
Prostatic urethra

Membranous urethra
Penile urethra
Corpus cavernosum penis

Corpus spongiosum penis

Glans penis
Testis
Epididymis
Scrotum

Bulbourethral gland and duct

Rectum
Seminal vesicle and duct
Ejaculatory duct
Prostate gland

B.   Median sagittal section through pelvis viewed from left

**FIGURE 1.3.** The male reproductive system.

**Source:** Eva Lurie Weinreb, *Anatomy and Physiology* (Reading, MA: Addison-Wesley Publishing, 1984), p. 778.

## Anus

The male anus, just like the female anus, is a highly erotic area. In fact, studies on anal stimulation and penetration of men reported by Shere Hite in *The Hite Report on Male Sexuality* (Ballantine, 1981) found that men truly enjoyed the experience. When stimulated there by heterosexual partners using a finger, many men reported that the orgasm was "physically exquisite." Ms. Hite stated that "the reason for this was probably due to the proximity of the prostate gland." Sexologists report that when manipulated properly, the prostate gland is highly erotic and can contribute to intense orgasms. To manipulate the prostate properly, Ms. Hite says that, with a finger inside the anal canal, one should press against the anterior wall of the anus and down slightly to locate the prostate. The prostate is about one inch in diameter and, according to Ms. Hite, continued stimulation of it can bring on orgasm. The manipulation should be sensual, not forceful.

## Cowper's Glands

The pea-sized Cowper's glands are located on the urethra, right below the prostate gland. Also known as the bulbourethral glands, the Cowper's glands produce the fluid or dripping men may experience when highly aroused. The mucuslike fluid is responsible for keeping the urethra well lubricated. The alkaline nature of this fluid neutralizes the acidic nature of any urine left in the urethra. This helps protect the sperm that are about to be ejaculated down the urethra.

*Note:* As just stated, the fluid from the Cowper's glands congregates on the head of the penis. Some sperm may be present right before ejaculation. It is possible, then, for a woman to become impregnated if her partner inserts his penis in her vagina before ejaculation actually takes place.

## Epididymis

The epididymis is a mass of tiny tubes connected to the testes. It is here where the sperm mature. The tubes within the epididymis merge to form the vas deferens, which serves as the passageway for the sperm. The epididymis also removes from storage those spermatozoa that are less likely to survive and destroys them.

## Glans

The glans, as stated, is the head of the penis. At the center of the glans is the small opening of the urethra. As in women, this is were the urine exits the body. It is also the tube through which semen is expelled from the body during ejaculation.

## Nipples

As in women, the nipples located on the chests of males become erect during sexual stimulation. Masters and Johnson discovered in their research that men under 60 years of age very seldom ejaculate without this obvious turgidity.

## Scrotum

At the base of the penis, you will find the bag of skin or pouch that houses the oval-shaped bodies known as the testicles. Within the scrotum are muscles and tissues that act like a yo-yo. Under normal circumstances, the temperature of the scrotum is just slightly lower than the general body temperature. When exposed to cold, the scrotum draws up to get extra heat. When the temperature is too warm, it drops down somewhat to cool off. This built-in natural mechanism is necessary for proper sperm production, which occurs at a slightly lower temperature. This is why the testes are outside of the body instead of inside, as the ovaries are in women. Nature is always working hard, doing the right thing!

## Perineum

The perineum is a very erotic sex zone. In men, it is located between the anus and the scrotum. During the orgasmic phase, when the testes and the scrotum rise toward and rest snug against the perineum, stimulating this area can bring on ejaculation.

## Seminal Vesicles

The seminal vesicles, located just behind the prostate, are the glands that make the bulk of the semen. The prostate gland, which wraps around the urethra and is found right below the bladder, produces a small amount of milky fluid that combines with the semen. Within this fluid are sugar, vitamins, minerals, and enzymes. These nutrients are responsible for helping to nourish and keep the sperm healthy. Every 4 grams of this fluid contains about 36 calories. It is a misconception that this ejaculate will cause weight gain when ingested.

James H. Gilbaugh Jr., M.D., one the country's leading urologists and the author of *A Doctor's Guide to Men's Private Parts* (Crown, 1989), reminds us that, contrary to popular belief, the testicles are not the major source of ejaculate fluid. Rather, the seminal vesicles manufacture about 70 percent of the ejaculate fluid that is expelled during the orgasmic phase. The prostate gland contracts at the height of sexual excitement and helps provide the force that causes the ejaculate to be expelled from the penis.

## Testicles

The oval-shaped testicles reside in the scrotum, the saclike pouch that hangs down below the penis. The testicles are comparable to the female ovaries. They produce sperm and the male sex hormone testosterone. Testosterone is what gives men their physical prowess and male characteristics. Estrogen, produced by the ovaries, is what gives women their female characteristics. Sperm are actually part of the fluid known as semen, or seminal fluid. When ejaculated into the vagina, they make their way toward the cervix to unite with the female egg. This union, known as fertilization, leads to pregnancy and the formation of a child.

## Urethra

The urethra is a tube that originates at the bladder and through which the urine travels to exit the body. It is also the tube through which the ejaculate travels. As you know, urine and semen cannot travel through the urethra at the same time. This is because an alkaline fluid is secreted into the urethra by the Cowper's glands. This fluid lubricates the urethra and neutralizes its acidity to allow the sperm to pass through unharmed.

## Vas Deferens

The vas deferens actually is a continuation of the epididymis, says Allen B. Weisse, M.D., a professor of medicine at the New Jersey Medical School in Newark. Dr. Weisse explains that the vas deferens transports the sperm from the epididymis just before ejaculation. The vas deferens runs just behind the bladder and joins with the excretory ducts of the seminal vesicles to form the ejaculatory ducts. It is the vas deferens that is tied off during the surgical birth-control procedure known as a vasectomy.

# 2

# The Biological Basis of Sexual Desire

*When the woman feels ready, she can hold the erect penis at an angle of about 45 degrees, pointed toward her partner's head, and slide down on it, letting her vagina snuggle around its head without attempting to insert it any farther. (See Figure 2.1.) Once in this position, resist the urge to start thrusting right away. Note the sensations you both are receiving, by establishing a quicker, shallower, thrusting pattern for a while. Women find this especially sensual, since nerve endings in the vagina are more heavily concentrated in the outer portion of the vagina than deep inside.*

William H. Masters, M.D., and
Virginia E. Johnson, D.Sc.
*Heterosexuality* (HarperCollins, 1994)

When you viewed the illustration and read the passage by the famed researchers of human sexuality Masters and Johnson, did you notice a sudden change in your breathing pattern? Was your breathing more pronounced or were your breaths short and shallow? Did your level of awareness seem to heighten? Were you suddenly focused on a sexual encounter of your own? Did your energy levels seem to peak just a little? Additionally, what changes did you sense in your reaction time, in your genital area, in your body temperature, and in your excitement level?

If you felt any of these changes after reading the passage, in a nutshell

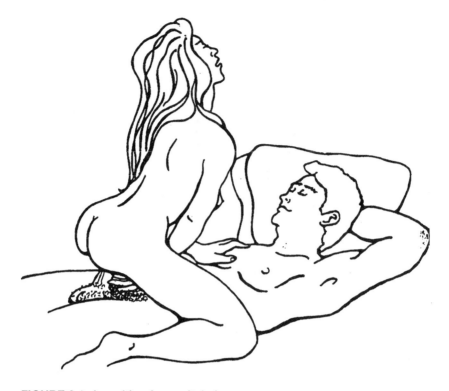

**FIGURE 2.1.** A position for genital play.

**Source:** William Masters, Virginia Johnson, and Robert Kolodny, *Heterosexuality* (New York: HarperCollins, 1994), p. 38.

you entered the "prime-time zone." When we are sexually aroused, our bodies go through a number of changes that heighten our senses and awareness. The changes also prepare us and motivate us to act on these impulses. Where do the impulses originate, and what causes the sudden rush of warm feelings, the fluctuation in body temperature, and the changes in body chemistry? Theresa L. Crenshaw, M.D., the author of *The Alchemy of Love and Lust* (G.P. Putnam's Sons, 1996), states that there is a whole battalion of substances flowing in our arteries and veins that are responsible for the changes that occur when we are sexually aroused.

In Chapter 2, we will take a look at this elaborate arsenal of weapons that throw our system into this frenzied state. We also will review the role the brain plays and the new research concerning these magical, mystical substances to which Dr. Crenshaw eludes that are called hormones.

# What Are Hormones?

Hans Selye, M.D., known as the father of stress research, stated in his book *Stress Without Distress* (Lippincott and Crowell, 1974) that:

> The apparent cause of illness is often an infection, an intoxication, nervous exhaustion or merely old age, but actually a breakdown of the hormonal adaptation mechanism appears to be the most common ultimate cause of death in man.

This is powerful stuff! And from the statement by Dr. Selye, it becomes obvious that hormones have something to do with regulating the metabolic actions and reactions within the human body. Robert A. Wallace, Ph.D., a professor at the University of Florida and author of *Biology: The World of Life* (Scott Foresman and Company, 1990), defines a hormone as a chemical messenger that is transmitted in body fluids from one part of an organism to another to produce a specific effect on the target cells and that regulates physiology, growth, differentiation, or behavior.

Based on our discussion thus far, a hormone could be compared to the postal service. You, the sender, mail a package across the country addressed to a specific location. The mail carrier delivers your package to your specified address, where the receiver of the package opens it and follows the instructions you included on how to properly operate the item you sent. In turn, the receiver sends you back a thank-you note (feedback) to let you know how things turned out.

So, as you can see, hormones are sent into tissue fluid and the bloodstream to be whisked away to all different parts of the body. These hormones do not actually participate in producing energy, but act as traffic cops, ensuring that the metabolic regulatory operations know when to start and stop.

# The Command Post

Dr. Ruth Westheimer, noted sex therapist, adamantly declares that one of the most powerful aphrodisiacs known is the one between the ears—the brain. Aphrodisiacs are substances ingested or applied to jump-start sexual arousal. We have implied that hormones are chemical messengers, with instructions for a target organ or cell. But where do the messages originate and how do the target cells, tissues, or organs read those messages?

As you might have surmised from Dr. Westheimer's belief, these signals originate in the brain. The gland located in the brain that is responsible for all this activity is the pituitary gland. The pituitary is known as the master gland because it releases hormones that signal other glands to secret hormones in response to bodily needs. For example, the pituitary signals the thyroid gland (located in the throat area) to release hormones that control the body's metabolic rate, which determines how efficiently we utilize food for energy, controls body weight (burns fat for energy), and performs a host of other functions.

The pituitary gland also discharges hormonal messengers that signal the sex glands, or gonads (the testes in males and the ovaries in females), to get to work. The gonads are where the host of hormones reside that drive most of our sexual desire. The hypothalamus gland in the brain controls the pituitary gland.

The adrenal glands are also involved in this messenger system. The adrenals are two small glands located atop the kidneys. They have two parts—an inner portion called the medulla and an outer portion called the cortex. The adrenals help us counter the effects of stress and produce hormones known as excitatory chemicals. These hormones, epinephrine (adrenaline) and norepinephrine, secreted by the adrenal medula, prepare and keep us "ready for action." Small amounts of the sex hormones estrogen and testosterone are also secreted by the adrenal cortex. It is important to remember, however, that the gonads are the primary producers of these hormones.

## A Quantum Leap

In his discussion of mind-body healing, Dr. Deepak Chopra reminds us that current thinking and data reveal that the mind and the body are connected and not separate entities, as once believed. Past scientific models proposed that we were physical machines that learned how to think. Dr. Chopra insists that the new quantum physics proposes a different model. In fact, he states that emerging science shows us that the opposite exists. Instead of being physical machines that have learned how to think, Dr. Chopra maintains that "we may be thoughts or quantum events in the field of information and energy that have learned how to create the physical machine."

Dr. Chopra also says we now know that the mind is not just confined to the brain, but exists in our cells, in our organs, and throughout our bodies. He goes one step further and suggests that this thinking mind is everywhere and exists everywhere, transcending the body, not simply localized within us.

What does this have to do with sex? Everything! As we move forward, you will see how you actually have some control over modulating how well your army of sexual motivators works for you today and in the future. Understanding how internal messages are sent and read is vital to understanding your sexual response and how to stay within your prime response zone for life.

## The Human Sexual Response

While there are many different hormonal systems that control our blood sugar, our metabolism, our internal water balance, and the calcium levels of our blood and bones, to name a few, all of these systems have a common denominator. That commonality has to do with what scientists call target tissues and receptor sites.

Researchers now know that receptor sites are on the surfaces of cells throughout the body. These sites can be compared to docks where ships and other vessels park. In the case of a ship or other vessel, it can refuel and carry out other activities while docked. In the case of our cells, hormones can transmit their messages to the target tissues or cells. Sexually speaking, the message to the testicles or ovaries would be to start pumping out more testosterone or estrogen, respectively, in preparation for an ensuing sexual encounter. This elaborate communication system between the mind and the body involving the hormonal systems is shown in Figure 2.2.

In the illustration, according to R. C. Khurana, M.D., a clinical assistant professor of medicine at the University of Pittsburgh School of Medicine, a plus-sign next to a hormone or body part indicates that the hormone or body part initiates or enhances the activity of a particular hormone. A minus-sign indicates that a hormonal messenger tells the hormone or body part to cease its activity.

This is referred to as a negative feedback system or loop. Hormone-

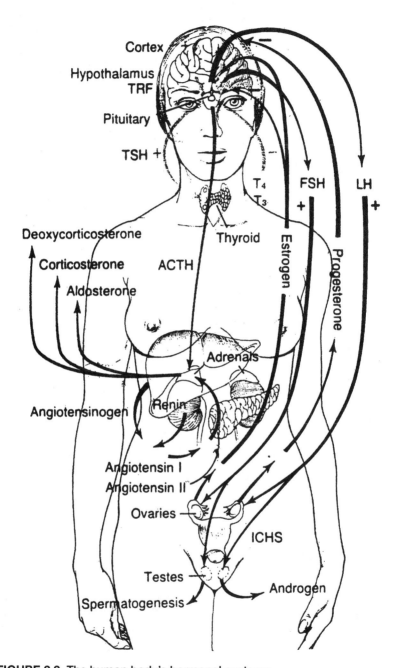

**FIGURE 2.2.** The human body's hormonal systems.

**Source:** R. C. Khurana, *You and Your Hormone Glands* (Pittsburgh: Obesity and Diabetes Books Publishing, 1978), p. 4.

producing glands, or endocrine glands, such as the adrenal, thyroid, and pituitary, are regulated by this negative feedback system. In many cases, according to Ruth L. Memmler, M.D., a professor emeritus of nursing at East Los Angeles College, the endocrine glands tend to oversecrete their hormones into the target tissues to ensure a strong effect. However, this can have a negative effect on the intended target tissues, so another message is sent out to decrease the secretory activity. This prevents over-stimulation of the gland.

So, in reality, sex is definitely more than just a contact sport. It should be easy to understand now why Dr. Westheimer suggests that the brain is the most powerful component of your sexual machinery.

For a moment, please think about how many times a day you become aroused. Think about the intensity of your arousal, how it subsides, and how it can then pulsate again. You have, as you can see, a built-in biological arsenal designed to meet the demands of your human sexual response. While estrogen and testosterone are the key players in this wild and frenzied melee, other hormones also play a part in the rise and fall of your sexual desire. Some of these hormones can make you feel like Tony the Tiger; others, like the Energizer Bunny, who keeps going and going; and still others, as calm and collected as James Bond.

## The Sex Brigade

Like most things in life, most of our hormonal systems use the checks-and-balances method. However, some of our hormones are released on a cyclic basic. For example, the hormones that control menstruation in women are released in a certain order each month. Other hormones surge at certain times, based on our emotional responses, our stress levels, our biological clock, or the natural rhythms of nature, such as day, night, or the seasons. For example, testosterone flows and peaks about every 15 to 20 minutes in males, while estrogen in females ebbs and flows in tune with various rhythmic cycles.

Let's take a look at the elite force of internal marauders that reminds us how pleasurable sex is, making us pursue it, want it, flaunt it, and, most important, maintain our biological capacity to continue our pursuit of it!

## DHEA

"DHEA" is short for "dehydroepiandrosterone." This hormone is made by the adrenal glands and is known as the youth hormone. DHEA rises at a constant rate into our twenties, then declines gradually after the age of 30. While DHEA is responsible for modulating a number of systems that deter aging, it is also linked to the sex drive, orgasms, and sexual appetite.

## Dopamine

Dopamine is the hormone primarily responsible for sexual desire. Like parents guiding and prodding their offspring toward excellence, dopamine propels us and commands us to pursue pleasure in general. This brain chemical could be called the anticipation molecule because it reminds us of pleasurable feelings, locks those feelings in our database, and pushes us to relive them over and over again.

## Estrogen

Known as the female hormone, estrogen is what gives women their female characteristics, including their hourglass figures and the physical softness that heightens and enhances their sex appeal. Estrogen, while found in both sexes, is predominant in women and regulates what health professionals call the receptive sex drive.

## Oxytocin

Oxytocin is known as the touching hormone because it is responsible for that bright red flush or glow we get when we touch or engage in sexual contact. Oxytocin heightens the pleasurable sensations of orgasm and bonds us to our loved ones.

## Phenylethylamine

Phenylethylamine (PEA) is a messenger hormone that makes us do those weird and wacky things we often do in the name of love. Known as the molecule of love, PEA really kicks in during the orgasmic phase. It makes us miss our partner and is associated with our yearning for him or her.

## Pheromones

Pheromones are invisible, odorless substances that are involved in sexual attraction. Human pheromones are marketed in the form of colognes, sprays, gels, and other products. These products have been shown in various trials to be connected to an increase in sexual activity by the individuals using them. For more information on pheromones, see page 143.

## Progesterone

Progesterone slows down and cools off the sex drive. It also is responsible for preparing and maintaining the lining of the uterus for pregnancy. While progesterone is critical to female well-being, it is vital to men's health. It is the primary precursor of adrenal cortical hormone and testosterone. Males utilize a lot less of this hormone than women do, but as they age, it becomes much more important to them as it helps balance their increasing levels of estrogen. It is important to remember that men and women have exactly the same hormones, only in differing amounts.

## Prolactin

Prolactin is known as the nurturing hormone because it stimulates the secretion of milk by the mammary glands. Prolactin peaks during the latter part of pregnancy and dulls the sensual feelings.

## Serotonin

Serotonin is a brain chemical that received much press a few years ago because of the diet pill fen-phen. Fen-phen heightened the effects of serotonin, which makes us feel cool, calm, and collected. Serotonin is the brain chemical that brings us back down to earth. When things get too heated, serotonin puts on the brakes to douse the flames. According to Dr. Theresa Crenshaw, low levels of serotonin can push the sex drive into overdrive and tend to cause both males and females to have orgasms very quickly.

## Testosterone

Known as an androgen hormone, testosterone is considered a male hormone. The opposite of estrogen, testosterone can be called the "go get 'em" hormone. It is responsible for the way we run, walk, skip, or jump in our pursuit of sex. Because testosterone enhances the brain chemical dopamine, it keeps our pedal to the metal in our pursuit of sexual gratification.

## Vasopressin

Vasopressin helps put the brakes on mounting levels of testosterone to ensure that sexual encounters are pleasurable. It heightens our perception and concentration, thus keeping sexual gratification in the prime-time zone.

# The Biological Nature of Desire

When you take a closer look at the larger picture, as described earlier by Dr. Chopra, it is evident that the biological aspects of our sexual desire were meant to be reciprocal. The internal communication system of checks and balances perpetuates life in general as well as our physical selves in particular and maintains the integrity of the larger information-and-energy system within and outside ourselves to which Dr. Chopra eludes. This is the true nature of our sexual desire, our pursuit of it, and the inborn communication system that ensures our pursuit is enjoyable, fulfilling, and permanent.

In the next chapter, "Forever Sexual," we will explore the concept of aging and the misconceptions that exist concerning sexual desire, abstinence, and the psychological and sociological aspects of maintaining sexual health.

# 3

# Forever Sexual

*Is sex after 50 an unnatural act, a vestigal (no longer present or of use) remnant designed by nature only for those of reproductive age? Or is sex a life-quality issue, a central function to be protected and cherished, like breathing or eating? Sex is very close to the essence of life. Some biologists claim that it is all there is to life.*

Walter M. Bortz II, M.D.
*Clinical Associate Professor of Medicine,*
*Stanford University School of Medicine*

Before we discuss the major topics of this chapter, I would like to ask you a few questions:

- Is your sex life emotionally rewarding and physically satisfying?
- Is it supercharged with excitement, versatility, imagination, and passion?
- Do you engage in sexual contact or intercourse two to four times a week?
- Are you 20 to 40 years of age?
- Do you understand and appreciate the fact that sex is for life?
- Are you sexually fit and knowledgeable about your approaching sexual life stages and those of your partners?

If you answered yes to any of the above questions, I would like to ask you one more question: How would you like to give up this part of your life?

I think I already know the answer to this last question. For the overwhelming majority of us, the thought of losing our sexual prowess, attractiveness, and skills is not only a frightening thought, but would be a devastating blow to our self-esteem and ego.

Walter M. Bortz II, M.D., clinical associate professor of medicine at Stanford University School of Medicine, maintains that sex is very close to the essence of life. Dr. Bortz, in his research, has found that when individuals, whether male or female, lose their sexual capabilities, they begin to disengage from society, their environment, their love ones, and, ultimately, themselves.

William Regelson, M.D., a professor of medicine at the Medical College of Virginia in Richmond, states that "many researchers feel that the essence of youth—indeed, the essence of feeling fully alive—is libido." Dr. Regelson calls this sexual stage the "youthful state" or "youthful advantage." It is in this stage, according to Dr. Regelson, that the ability to be stimulated and aroused by the environment is often the key to remaining youthful. This is why he believes that remaining sexually active is so important.

The esteemed sex researchers Bernard D. Starr, Ph.D., and Marcella Bakur Weiner, Ed.D., go a step further, noting that sex is a psychological as well as a physical need. These two eminent scientists claim that it is through our sexual contact with others that we heal emotional scars, soothe anger, express joy, and claim redemption. Dr. Starr and Dr. Weiner, in their investigations of human sexuality, found that these emotions and the need to express them via sexual contact is a life-long one.

*Are we really capable of having and enjoying sexual contact well into our seventies, eighties, and nineties?* According to past and present experts on human sexuality, yes we are!

For example, Joseph Poticha, M.D., assistant clinical professor of obstetrics-gynecology at the Chicago Medical School, says:

> One of the biggest surprises I got in my early years as a doctor was the discovery that people in their 60's, 70's, even 80's and beyond could continue to have sex. The prospect of being able to have it virtually all my life was a happy one.

Morris Notelovitz, M.D., Ph.D., president and medical director of the Women's Medical and Midlife Centers of America in Gainesville, Florida, says:

Although both men and women experience a decline in sexual responsiveness as they grow older, there's no physiological reason why you can't continue to enjoy sex throughout the middle years and beyond.

Alex Comfort, M.D., a well-known sexologist and the author of *The Joy of Sex* (Crown, 1991), states that "the first step in preserving your sexuality, which for many people is deeply important in preserving personhood, is to realize that, if cultivated, sexuality can be, and normally is, lifelong, for both sexes." Dr. Comfort is saying that sexual function can be a long-term activity *if it is cultivated*. As we learned in Chapter 2, sex is a biological function that nature intended to be a life-long experience. It also becomes evident when viewing sexuality from this biological standpoint that the ability to remain sexually healthy—that is, to preserve your inborn sexual mechanisms and responses—does not exist in a vacuum. By this I mean your future sexuality may be biologically assured, but in reality, it is not impervious to the ravages of time, the environment, disease, and, in many cases, lifestyle.

If you are within the age range mentioned at the beginning of this chapter, you must recognize that according to current data, you still have anywhere from 20 to 60 years left *sexually*. Make no mistake about it: Whether you are male or female, your sexuality is an important part of your future health.

## We Are Sexual Beings

Richard Green, M.D., professor of psychiatry and behavioral sciences at the State University of New York at Stony Brook and editor of *Human Sexuality: A Health Practitioner's Text* (Williams and Wilkins, 1979), states: "Emotional health and physical health are so interwoven that neglect of the emotional is neglect of the physical. Sexual health is so integral to both that to ignore the sexual is poor patient care."

When you view human sexuality from this purely biological viewpoint, it is easy to understand why researchers insist that we were designed to have life-long sexual capabilities. This has been ensured by nature via the elaborate system of checks and balances installed within us. This system guarantees nature's continued perpetuation of itself. Within the larger context of this continuum, we serve as energy-filled power plants with an endless supply of sexual information that signals and directs this uninterrupted process of arousal and interaction with the environment that surrounds us.

Carlon M. Colker, M.D., a physician with Beth Israel Medical Center in New York and author of *Sex Pills: From Androstenedione to Zinc* (Advanced Research Press, 1999), also maintains that life exists for no other reason than to reproduce itself. He says that this was and continues to be too simple a concept for us to accept. Dr. Colker, however, reminds us that within the context of this assumption, our human need to seek and fulfill our sexual desires clearly outweighs our need to procreate, which in reality actually supersedes nature's intentions.

## Understanding That Sexuality Lasts Forever

One of the most profound myths about aging and sexual capabilities is that sexual dysfunction is inevitable. Dr. Bortz, also the author of *Dare to Be 100* (Simon & Schuster, 1996) and a leading expert in the field of health and aging, notes that throughout our life cycle, we lose only .5 percent of our bodily functions per year statistically. According to Dr. Bortz, a person 65 years of age has lost only 15 percent of his or her vitality, energy, or life-force mechanisms. Dr. Bortz maintains that the majority of our most important phsysiological functions are intact and operational throughout our life and up to the time of our death.

Once you realize this fact, it becomes evident why modern-day researchers insist that our sexual potential is boundless. It is connected to the energy-filled information system that sustains life and nature itself. Sex is a vital part of this universal communication system. In more practical terms, our emotions, our physical makeup, our sexual characteristics, our wants and desires, are all interwoven in this infinite cycle of ubiquitous events that sustain, support, and prolong life.

Somewhere, right this minute, human sexual contact is being made, joyfully, emotionally, and, in many cases, with vivid imagination and spontaneity. This human emotion is part of every person's life continuum within the larger context of nature's continuum. Each one of us has the capacity to enjoy this extraordinary, sensory-filled expression forever, as nature intended. Cultivation, however, is the key to protecting and preserving this powerful, interminable "orgasmic force" we call sex.

## The Invisible Hand of Nature

To reiterate, while sexual decline may be associated with aging, it is not inevitable. Dr. Howard Peiper and Nina Anderson, authors of *Natural Solutions for Sexual Dysfunction* (Safe Goods, 1998), remind us that if nothing is done to slow down the natural mechanisms of aging, sexual dysfunction can occur. The facts are that aging does cause a decline of the hormonal levels in both men and women. According to Peiper and Anderson, this can cause an array of problems that, if left unchecked, can threaten your potential to remain sexually fit for life.

However, many sexual-health researchers, such as Leslie R. Schover, Ph.D., a professor and clinical psychologist in sexual rehabilitation at the M. D. Anderson Hospital of the Texas Medical Center in Houston, say that aging, even old age, is not the problem in reference to sexual decline. For the most part, Dr. Schover argues that many of the problems associated with sexual dysfunction are caused by the diseases that sometimes occur later in life, such as diabetes, arteriosclerosis (hardening of arteries), and kidney damage. Heavy smoking, drinking, surgeries to the pelvic area, and medication to control high blood pressure also are the real culprits, she says. The key question then becomes: How do we preserve, manage, and cultivate our life-long sexual potential?

Before we can answer this question, we need to have a working knowledge of common complaints in reference to sexual dysfunction. And keep in mind that "sexual dysfunction" simply means that *something ain't working right*. In Part II of this book, we will take a close look at sexual decline, or actually, changes in our natural sexual self. We will look at both male and female sexual disorders and at the forces behind many forms of sexual disturbances.

Once you have a better understanding of the common complaints related to aging, it becomes easier to find answers to the questions above. In many cases, you will find that you have some waning of your sexual abilities, but that for the most part, *the hardest thing to do is protect your body from yourself!*

# PART II

# WHEN DESIRE
# TAKES
# A HOLIDAY

*Lack of desire is not one single condition, but a group of illnesses with different causes that share common symptoms.*

Waguih R. Guirguis, M.D.
*Director, Psychosexual Clinic,
St. Clement's Hospital, Ipswich, England*

- When was the last time you had knock 'em down, bang 'em up, ring-a-ding-ding sex?
- When was the last time you had a loving, soulful, sensual, and passionate session that did not necessarily focus on sexual intercourse?
- When was the last time you planned an evening with the intent to heighten, improve, explore, or rekindle lost sexual desire?
- When was the last time you fantasized about an unforgettable sexual experience?
- When was the last time you used a self-stimulative method to pleasure yourself sexually?
- When was the last time you initiated sex with your partner?
- When was the last time you dressed yourself provocatively to entice your sexual partner?
- When was the last time you were turned on sexually when seeing someone you found very attractive?
- How many times in the last several weeks have you avoided sexual contact with your partner?
- Have you found that erotic movies, sexual devices, and even self-manipulation methods fail to stimulate you sexually?
- Has sex become a chore rather than an outlet or expression of your sexuality?
- Has sex become an afterthought?

If you are 20, 30, 40, 50, or even 60 years old or beyond and suffer from a general lack of sexual desire, you are not alone. It is estimated that more than 20 million women and men suffer from the malady known as *hypoactive sexual desire disorder, sexual arousal disorder, inhibited sexual desire, desire phase dysfunction,* or *inhibited sexual excitement,* all interchangeable terms.

What has changed in your life? How did you get to this point? Lack of sexual desire, as stated by Dr. Guirguis on page 39, is not a single condition but rather a group of illnesses with different causes that share common symptoms. This is the focus of the next two chapters "Female Sexual Disorders" and "Male Sexual Disorders." In these chapters, we will take a look at some of the most common problems associated with sexual dysfunction. Additionally, we will review many of the machines and devices that are used to compensate for the loss of sexual capabilities. Niels Lauersen, M.D., a diplomate of the American Board of Obstetrics and Gynecology, insists that "despite all the openness and understanding in the world there are sexual problems or dysfunctions that have complex causes." According to Dr. Lauersen, many, such as frigidity, vaginismus, impotency, and premature ejaculation, are linked in some cases to severe psychological or emotional factors. These dysfunctions can result in the complete shutdown of an individual's sexual communication system, thus interfering with the ability to enjoy or in many cases even engage in sexual coitus or copulation.

What forces are behind this downward spiral? Can they be controlled or slowed down? Are they inevitable? If we have the ability to remain sexually active and healthy for life, why are so many people sexually dysfunctional? Answering these questions and others related to the loss of one's inborn sexual capabilities is the focus of Part II of this book.

When desire takes a holiday, the emotional and psychological ramifications can be devastating. One of the most powerful and provocative feelings we have as humans is that of responding to sexual stimuli. Sexual desire is an intricate part of the human experience. However, lack or loss of it is not part of the normal or evolutional process of human development or existence.

As already discussed, healthcare professionals now know that the variables surrounding sexual decline are not all related to aging and declining hormone levels. Lifestyle choices may play a more important role in accelerating sexual decline than previously thought. Additionally, the outdated prognosis of it being all in your head is no longer accepted as final. New methods of treatment and testing are now available. Suffering in silence is no longer an option you have to choose.

# 4

# Female Sexual Disorders

*The basic problem in orgasmic impairment is that the brain
and vagina are not reliably connected to each other. It is like
a telephone with loose wires. Sometimes the line goes dead
in the middle of a conversation, sometimes the message is
garbled in the process and sometimes the phone doesn't
even ring.*

David Reuben, M.D.
*Everything You Always Wanted
to Know About Sex*
(St. Martin's Press, 2000)

Dr. Alfred Kinsey in his landmark study on female sexuality, *Sexual
Behaviors in the Human Female* (W.B. Saunders Company, 1953), found
that women reach their sexual peak in their late twenties or during their
thirties. According to Dr. Kinsey, women generally remain at this plateau through their sixties, after which they may show a slight decline in
sexual response capability. This finding by Dr. Kinsey completely con-
tradicts the above comment by Dr. David Reuben. Dr. Kinsey believed
that women have the capability of enjoying and responding to sexual
stimuli well into their twilight years. In fact, sexual health professionals
maintain that women at age 60 are still capable of having multiple orgasms. However, the lack of sensory feelings commonly known as
frigidity affects millions of women in varying age groups. As a point of
reference here, the *Merck Manual of Diagnosis and Therapy* (Merck
and Company, 1999) defines frigidity, or *inhibited sexual excitement*, as

recurrent and persistent inhibition of sexual excitement during sexual activity, manifested by partial or complete failure to attain the lubrication and swelling response of sexual excitement or to maintain it until completion of the sexual act. The editors of this highly respected medical manual insist that this inhibition actually occurs despite what clinical therapists deem to be adequate sexual stimulation in focus, intensity, and duration.

Dr. Reuben, on the contrary, believes that many women while engaging in sexual intercourse do not experience any of the associated pleasurable sensations. This problem, also known as inhibited sexual arousal, is one of the most common sexual disorders women have, according to a study published in the *Journal of the American Medical Association* in February 1999. In this study, women cited loss of sex drive or desire as their number one problem concerning sexuality, followed by lack of arousal and pain during sexual intercourse.

Female sexual dysfunction disorders are usually classified as desire, arousal, orgasmic, or pain disorders. Painful sexual coitus is further divided into the two general classifications of dyspareunia and vaginismus. In this chapter, we will review these disorders.

## Low Sexual Desire and Arousal

Low sexual desire and arousal can be compared to impotency or erectile dysfunction in males. Females who experience these losses of sensory expression generally do so consistently and on a regular basis. Females who aren't sexually aroused are not just feeling fatigued or having a bad day, a headache, or a problem associated with premenstrual syndrome (PMS). One former and very attractive female client of mine once compared this phenomenon to being deaf. What was frustrating to this client was her ability to initiate or provoke a powerful and profound sexual response in her partner, but to never be able to enjoy the physical pleasures elicited by her physical beauty.

Like males who experience psychological problems owing to the inability to sustain an erection, many women eventually begin to find ways to avoid sexual contact, as the experience begins to become unpleasant and a very unintimate situation.

The whole group of disorders including decreased sex drive, low libido, and diminishing sexual excitement is now classified under the heading of FSAD. FSAD stands for female sexual arousal disorder. At a recent international conference on female sexual dysfunction, FSAD was defined as the persistent or recurrent inability to attain or maintain sufficient sexual excitement, causing personal distress. According to the distinguished panel of sexual health experts attending the conference from across the globe, the distress usually orginates because of diminished arousal, failure of genital lubrication, or another response associated with sexual stimuli.

Like chronic fatigue and premenstrual syndrome, FSAD has caused women to suffer humiliation, denial, and the common diagnosis that "it's all in your head." This trend, however, is changing thanks to modern-day pioneers such as Dr. Jennifer Berman and Dr. Laura Berman.

The disorder is now recognized as a condition that warrants further study and research. It usually manifests itself in one or more of the following symptoms:

- Inability to reach orgasm
- Decreased libido
- Lack of clitoral sensation
- Inadequate lubrication
- Painful intercourse
- Disinterest in having sexual intercourse

Researchers cite many reasons for the loss of sensation in the genital area. Improper blood flow to the sexual organs, traumatic sexual experience, conflict in the relationship (in 80 percent of cases), as well as many of the following reasons:

- Hormonal problems
- Adrenal disorders
- Insufficient production of estrogen or testosterone
- Pelvic injury
- Hypothyroidism (underactive thyroid)
- Vaginitis (inflamed vagina)
- Spinal cord injury
- Endometriosis (uterine disorder)
- Stress and anxiety
- Depression
- Hypertension (high blood pressure)
- Medication (antidepressant, high blood pressure, cholesterol lowering, tranquilizers, sedatives)
- Chronic pain disorder
- Birth control pills
- Aging and degenerative disease (arthritis, heart disease, diabetes)

- Fibroid tumors
- Yeast infection
- Urinary-tract infection
- Interstitial cystitis (chronic inflammation of the bladder)
- Pelvic floor prolapse (loss of firmness and elasticity of the connective tissue and muscles that hold the bladder, uterus, vagina, and rectum in place)
- Chronic fatigue
- Hysterectomy (removal of the uterus)
- Cervical cancer or removal of the cervix
- Vestibulitis (inflammation and/or burning sensation at the vaginal opening)
- Use of alcohol or illegal or illicit drugs
- Vaginismus (painful intercourse due to physical or emotional problems)

Also take, for example, the experience of one of my female colleagues who was battling the ill effects that fibroid tumors and endometriosis can have on female sexuality. When she approached her personal physician about her concerns over not being able to physically experience the pleasurable sensations and erotic thoughts that usually occur during coitus and orgasms, she was told she was having them—she just didn't know it.

It is this loss of sensual feelings that causes many females to lose interest in exploring their sexuality. The loss of sexual interest also often leads women to avoid intimate encounters whose purpose is to meet the sexual needs of their partners. This will without professional help and communication lead to relationship issues. Due to this, Masters and Johnson contended that sexual dysfunction is a two-person issue and should be treated as such.

## Inhibited Orgasmic Disorder

According to the editors of the *Merck Manual,* female patients' primary complaint concerning orgasm centers on the inability to become aroused. This coincides with the analogy of being deaf made by my former female client. The difference, of course, is being able to see and interact with your surroundings without hearing sound versus not being able to feel or sense pleasure as a result of interaction.

In their book *For Women Only* (Henry Holt and Company, 2001),

Dr. Jennifer Berman and Dr. Laura Berman tell of a patient's battle to overcome the inability to become aroused. The client, who was married, had not had an orgasm in three years. She described herself as being dead from the waist down. This derangement is known in clinical terms as inhibited orgasmic disorder. It is defined as a persistent or recurrent delay in or absence of orgasm following a normal sexual excitement phase. This disorder, much like erectile dysfunction or impotency in males, can put a severe strain on even the most solid relationship. Inhibited orgasmic disorder is a problem affecting women of varying age groups, social and economic status, and nationalities. It is just beginning to receive the attention it deserves.

## Treatment Options

Researchers today use a wide range of tests to assess the origins of sexual problems. The treatment modalities that follow are all used interchangeably to correct FSAD. Dr. Laura Berman initially employs a 45-minute psychosexual evaluation she created called the Biopsychosocial Sexual Evaluation System (BSES). This subjective survey is designed to get not only the sexual history of the patient, but also an initial impression of the source of the sexual function complaints, says Dr. Berman. Other problems like surgeries, drugs, spinal cord injuries, and hormonal problems are also evaluated to help decide on appropriate treatment.

In addition to treating any problems noted via the BSES, reteaching or introducing new methods of erotic stimulation are also considered in correcting desire, arousal, and orgasmic disorders.

### SPECIAL NOTE

With the success of Viagra (sildenafil), there are numerous trials going on to find out how well the drug works on women. As we have learned, women have the same erectile tissue as men and can suffer from the same obstruction of proper blood flow to the genital area as men.

One form of treatment that has been surrounded by much controversy is hormone therapy, specifically androgen therapy. In Chapter 1, we learned that the hormones estrogen and progesterone are dominant in women and have a powerful influence on female sexuality. We also discussed how women make appreciable amounts of testosterone, which is an androgen and the predominant hormone in males. Testosterone, just like estrogen, is manufactured in females by the ovaries and the adrenal glands. As in males, this androgen (a hormone that has the ability to build up) declines over the course of a lifetime. It is a known fact that a precipitous drop in this hormone can wreak havoc on a women's sex drive. For this reason many physicians today suggest not only the replacement of estrogen but testosterone too.

Susan Rako, M.D., author of *The Hormone of Desire: The Truth About Testosterone, Sexuality, and Menopause* (Harmony Books, 1996), claims that without testosterone, improving a women's sex drive and other problems associated with aging and waning hormonal levels is severely compromised. Morris Notelovitz, M.D., Ph.D., coauthor of *Menopause and Midlife Health* (St. Martin's Press, 1993), states that "low levels of androgens have been implicated with being a major causative factor in menopausal related symptoms such as depression, headaches, bone loss and low libido."

By bringing testosterone ranges up to normal levels (14 to 76 nanograms per deciliter of blood), many of the above complications can be corrected. The problem with this method is that high dosages may cause increased hair growth, masculine (male) features, and other side effects such as elevated cholesterol levels and an increased risk of heart and liver disease. When administering testosterone, doctors closely monitor patients to ensure these associated risks are kept to a minimum.

The Drs. Berman state, "To us, testosterone is so central to a woman's sexual function that no lover and no amount of sexual stimulation can make up for its absence." From her research Dr. Rako has found safe acceptable ranges to be 20 to 50 nanograms per deciliter of blood.

### SPECIAL NOTE

Many women who undergo estrogen replacement therapy (ERT) are unaware that taking estrogen without testosterone can actually cause testosterone levels to drop. This happens because a hormone known as steroid hormone binding globulin (SHBG) attaches to the testosterone present in the body, making its use by the body almost impossible.

Because of the above factors, many women find it necessary to also replace small amounts of their declining androgens in order to fully correct many of their problems related to diminished sex drive, arousal, lubrication, and orgasm. Some women need to begin doing this during perimenopause, the years just before menopause when parts of these problems often begin. The well-known author on women's health issues Gail Sheehy in her *New York Times* best-seller, *The Silent Passage: Menopause* (Pocket Books, 1993), states: "The vast majority of women have no idea they are in something called perimenopause. Yet a woman's attitude and awareness going into this momentous passage have a profound impact on how it is experienced."

Ms. Sheehy notes that the last person to whom most women talk about their sexual problems is their healthcare professional. By the time they do, says Ms. Sheehy, many women are often in a state of panic. This may be due to the fact that during this time period there can be as much as a 30 percent decline in the amount of androgens, namely testosterone, that the female body is producing. Judith Reichman, M.D., medical correspondent for the "Today" show and author of *I'm Not in the Mood: What Every Woman Should Know About Improving Her Libido* (William Morrow, 1998), says that testosterone deficiency has a global effect. She notes that females don't lose desire just for their partner, but for any partner, even Tom Cruise or Sean Connery.

In Part IV of this book we will examine many of the preventive measures, natural foods, and supplement programs that you may want to consider in attacking this problem.

## Painful Coitus

Painful sexual coitus falls into two categories: dyspareunia and vaginismus.

### Dyspareunia

Dyspareunia is the clinical name for painful intercourse. One of the primary reasons we avoid sex is lack of energy, stamina, and zest for life. The other is pain. Many of today's long-term degenerative diseases like arthritis and chronic fatigue syndrome dampen even the healthiest sex drive. Pain can be one of the most devastating deterrents to human sexuality. While "Not tonight, honey, I have a headache" has become the satirical reason for avoiding a partner's sexual advances, dyspareunia is a very real and frightening experience.

To be in pain is one thing, but to experience excruciating pain during and even after sexual intercourse can be very frustrating. Many women, due to declining estrogen levels and thinning vaginal wall linings, experience this. Dr. Reichman claims that this is the most common complaint reported to gynecologists. She insists that in up to 76 percent of the women who suffer from this condition, there is an underlying physical reason. However, according to Dr. Reichman, many physicians dismiss the problem as an "all in your head" malady. This may be because the initial examination may reveal that nothing is physically wrong. However, pain may be localized, just outside the vaginal barrel, or may happen only during deep penile thrusts. Pain can also be the result of some hidden infection. Or the problem could be lack of sufficient vaginal lubrication, a tumor, scarring from previous pelvic surgery, the aftereffects of rape, or inadequate foreplay. Many of the reasons given for desire, arousal, and orgasmic problems can also cause dyspareunia. Peter R. Kilmann, Ph.D., director of the Human Sexuality Project at the University of South Carolina, and colleagues maintain that the treatment for painful intercourse should be very similar to that for orgasmic problems and vaginismus.

## Vaginismus

Vaginismus is also characterized by painful intercourse and is considered less of a enigma than orgasmic dysfunction. However, it can cause psychological problems, which in many cases contribute to the disorder. Religious beliefs, antisexual lifestyles, sexual fears and lack of knowledge, as well as abuse or trauma can play a role in the manifestation of vaginismus.

Sexual intercourse or the insertion of objects such as tampons, fingers, or sexual stimulation toys or devices causes spasms to occur in all of the outer muscles of the vagina. About 12 to 17 percent of all women suffer from this condition. These spasms can be so intense that penile insertion into the vagina can become impossible. Many times the pain that accompanies sexual intercourse, or the anticipation of it, can trigger these spasmatic reactions.

Laura E. Corio, M.D., gynecologist at the Mount Sinai Medical Center, says that these spasms actually originate in the brain as a defense mechanism. The brain instructs vaginal muscles to contract with enough force to prevent penetration into the vagina. As you could imagine, this will eventually dampen both the woman's sexual desire as well as that of her partner. Treatment for this disorder involves both partners and includes psychological testing, relaxation techniques, and other methods.

In practical terms, it is a known fact that pain and sexual desire do not make good bedfellows.

In the next chapter, "Male Sexual Disorders," we will look at some of the problems experienced by men. That chapter is not only for men just as this chapter was not only for women. Sexual partners should educate one another. After all, when one partner's sexuality is compromised, so is the other's. Tackle your sexual problems head on, as a team, and you both will win.

# 5

# Male Sexual Disorders

*Concerns about male sexual functioning are focused almost
exclusively on impotence, ejaculatory problems, and loss of
desire for sex.*

Allen B. Weisse, M.D.
*The Man's Guide to Good Health*
(Consumer Reports Books, 1991)

Dr. Allen Weisse, cardiologist and professor of medicine at the New
Jersey Medical School in Newark, believes there are other complications
associated with male sexual dysfunction besides the three he mentions
above. There are, as you may already be aware, a number of physiological, anatomical, psychological, and, as with women, lifestyle factors
that can prevent males from having a pleasurable and fruitful sex life.
Consider a few of the examples below:

- AIDS
- Alcoholism
- Benign prosthetic hyperplasia
  (enlarged prostate gland)
- Blood vessel disease
- Constipation
- Degenerative diseases (diabetes,
  high blood pressure, arterio-
  sclerosis)

- Medications
- Obesity
- Orchitis (infection of the
  tesiticles)
- Performance anxiety
- Peyronie's disease (abnormal
  curvature of the penis)
- Prostatis (inflamed prostate
  gland)

- Depression
- Dyspareunia in the man's partner
- Dysuria (pain or burning when urinating)
- Genital herpes
- Heart disease
- Kidney disease
- Klinefelter's syndrome (endocrine disorder in which insufficient steroid hormones are produced to allow erections to occur)
- Priapism (prolonged erections without sexual stimuli, which may be a sign of blood disorder)
- Prostate cancer
- Radiation
- Spinal cord injury (nerve damage)
- Surgery (bladder, rectum, penile, testicular)
- Thyroid disease
- Unresolved relationship issues

While we cannot cover all of the possible disorders that relate to a male's sexual health, we will concentrate on the three common problems cited by Dr. Weisse.

## Impotency

Estimates indicate that there are more than 20 million men in America who suffer from impotency. In individual terms, one out of every eight men in the United States has problems maintaining, sustaining, or achieving an erection. David F. Mobley, M.D., and Steven K. Wilson, M.D., both board-certified urologists who specialize in erectile dysfunction (impotency), define this disorder as "a man's inability to gain or maintain an erection adequate enough for the completion of sexual intercourse." In their book *Reversing Impotence Forever!* (Swan Publishing, 1995), they note a fallacy many people have concerning impotency. Being impotent does not mean that a male is incapable of fathering children, ejaculating, having orgasms, or feeling sexual desire. The male who is impotent has, due to a number of different reasons, lost the ability to fill the penis with blood and/or prevent the leakage or backflow of blood into the chambers known as the corpora cavernosa. When this happens, erections cannot be sustained long enough to engage in sexual intercourse.

Males have long denied and tried to mask the overbearing feelings of failure when this happens. It is important to seek help; in many cases lifestyle changes can correct the situation. Impotency is a common problem that is associated with aging. In fact, sexual health experts contend that by age 60 at least 18 percent of all males in the United States suffer from some form of impotency. That number jumps to nearly 75 percent by age 80.

Dr. Mobley and Dr. Wilson state that "men who begin to show signs of impotency at times worry without reacting and doing something about the problem." They argue vehemently that impotency is treatable, but you must take action to correct it.

This is the major goal of *Sensual for Life*: to guide you in preparing a life-long plan of action to help your recognize possible problems and solve them without putting your health at risk. Break the code of silence. Seek help, react, and, most important, communicate your concerns to your partner and your healthcare professional.

We know that when males are stimulated sexually, the penis becomes erect and rigid. Not only can the inability to maintain an erection be psychologically devastating to the man, but it can have the same effect on his partner. Many females mistakenly consider the problem to be a loss of interest in their feminine attributes. Honest communication is important, just as reassurance from your partner is. It also is important for females to understand the biological processes that allow erection to occur. Impotency can be caused by many different factors. The scientific facts are that, biologically, males are capable of having and sustaining erections suitable enough to engage in sexual intercourse well into their nineties and beyond. Let's take a look at this process and find out what actually happens from a physiological and a psychological standpoint.

## How Erections Occur

Before we review the physiological and psychological mechanisms that cause erections to happen, let's first review what does not cause them to occur. Penile erections are not a result of a strong-minded individual hell-bent on having sexual intercourse. As a matter of fact, erections occur due to the orchestrated efforts of the brain, spinal cord, hormones, blood vessels, nervous system, heart, penile arteries, and corpus cavernosa.

When you view proper erectile function from this orchestrated standpoint, it becomes apparent that when one instrument of the ensemble is out of sync, nature's biological promise of potency is suddenly compromised. You cannot will, demand, or wish an erection to occur. In fact, as we will learn in more detail in the chapters that follow, a relaxed state of mind and a healthy body are crucial to maintaining and sustaining the ability to have strong, powerful erections throughout your lifetime.

As suggested earlier by Dr. Ruth Westheimer, the brain is the most powerful natural aphrodisiac you have. It is here where it all starts— your sexual desire, response, and appetite. Your thoughts about a sexual encounter cause messengers in your brain known as neurotransmitters to activate nerve centers that process your libidinous or titillating thoughts.

It is difficult at times for men to see themselves as a conglomeration of chemicals. You are part of the biological and physiological processes that cause the penis to become erect. One of the chemicals responsible for erections is nitric oxide. Nitric oxide is discharged in the corpora cavernosa during sexual stimulation, thus triggering the release of the enzyme guantylate cyclase, which causes the levels of cyclic guanosine menophosphate to rise. This last chemical is what causes the smooth muscles found in the corpora cavernosa of the penis to relax. This allows blood being pumped from the heart to flow into the penis. Actually, it is the corpora cavernosa that swell, transforming the penis from a placid (relatively inert, idle, and shy, so to speak) sexual organ to the strong, hard, erect, and responsive sexual organ nature preprogrammed it to be.

In addition to all the things that must happen from a psychological and physiological standpoint, Dr. Mobley and Dr. Wilson ask us to add the process of aging to the equation. "When you take all this into consideration," they state, "it is not surprising that impotency can and will occur in so many men." Additionally, Robert Fried, Ph.D., clinical director of the Stress and Biofeedback Clinic at the Albert Ellis Institute in New York City, and Woodson C. Merrell, M.D., assistant clinical professor at Columbia University, state that "given the complex nature of this biological process it's easy to see how erections might potentially be affected at a number of different stages."

Leslie R. Schover, Ph.D., assistant professor at the Sexual Rehabilitation Center of the M. D. Anderson Hospital at Texas Medical Center, says that "we have been taught that erection problems are unavoidable with age." She explains that while it is true that erectile dysfunction problems are more common as men age, recent studies imply that impotency is not part of the natural aging process. Dr. Schover has found that many men without certain risk factors, or in spite of them, continue to have full erections into their eighties and nineties.

## Diagnosing Erection Problems

While loss of the ability to have an erection can be devastating to the male ego, it is wise to seek professional assistance to make sure there are no underlying medical conditions that may be causing the problem. Sexual health professionals employ the use of a wide variety of tests to determine the possible cause of impotency. They will generally test your:

- Hormone levels, especially your testosterone levels
- Nerve response levels
- Voiding (urinary) habits
- Blood sugar levels (for diabetes)
- Thyroid function
- Psychological and emotional state
- Nighttime penile erections

Penile erections usually occur several times during the night in healthy males during rapid eye movement (REM) sleep cycles. REM sleep is our deepest and most relaxed state of sleep. Sex therapists have long used nighttime penile erections as a barometer to rule out possible physical causes of erectile dysfunction.

In fact, Richard Berger, M.D., assistant professor of urology at the University of Washington Medical School, says, "Researchers have found that men have about five to six erections during sleep." Dr. Berger explains that these nighttime erections can last in some cases up to 25 minutes each. Also, while health officials do not know why they occur (in the absence of erotic thoughts), they are believed to be nature's way of exercising the penis to ensure the erection process continues.

# Ejaculation Problems

Ejaculation is defined as the ejection of semen from the body. This process usually happens in two separate phases. The first is called the contractile, or emission, phase. During this phase the male prostate gland, which is a donut-shaped organ surrounding the urethra, compresses and expels semen into the urethra. During the second phase, known as the expulsion phase, semen is forced through the urethra like a rushing river and is ejected from the tip of the penis.

Arthur C. Guyton, M.D., professor and chairman of the Department of Physiology and Biophysics at the University of Mississippi School of Medicine, breaks the ejaculation process into the following steps:

1. When sexual stimulation has reached the height of arousal, nerve centers in the tip of the spinal cord send messages to the sympathetic nerves in the male genitals.
2. The testes begin to contract (rhythmic peristalsis), which eventually induces contractions in the seminal vesicles, the vas deferens, the epididymis, and the penis itself.
3. The contractions push the sperm all the way from the testes through the various glands to the tip of the penis, where it is expelled.

This explosive expression of orgasm is unique to the male. As a matter of fact, Masters and Johnson contend that the male and female responses to sexual stimuli up to and through the orgasmic phase are the same despite the anatomic differences between the two sexes, but ejaculation is common in the male while only possible in the female.

One of the major problems associated with the ejaculatory process in men is what sexual health authorities refer to as premature ejaculation. Individuals who suffer from this disorder may ejaculate well in advance of sexual intercourse or within seconds of contact with the female vagina.

Premature ejaculation is one of the most frustrating sexual dysfunctions (for both partners). It affects more than 10 million American men, according to the University of Toronto Sexual Education and Peer Counseling Center. While extensive research has been conducted into the etiology of this disorder, no definitive physical component has been found. Many sexual health therapists consider it to be psychological in origin, due to negative early sexual experience, performance anxiety, lack of sexual knowledge, or fear, guilt, or anxiety. To combat this disorder, sexual health professionals use a variety of techniques and methods. They include exercises to delay ejaculation, behavioral and sexual position changes, discussion of personal and interrelationship problems, and psychotherapy.

Another problem associated with the ejaculatory process is the inability to ejaculate without extensive sexual stimulation. As you can imagine, although this malady is rare, it can become the source of sexual tension and frustration between partners. Retrograde ejaculation some-times referred to as dry ejaculation occurs when the flow of semen trav-els backward into the bladder instead of forward to be ejected through the penis. This rarity is usually found in men who have had certain prostate surgical procedures performed. Ejaculation, to many couples, is highly stimulating, and retrograde ejaculation can cause mild to severe psychological trauma for both sexual partners.

Painful ejaculation for many males makes having, wanting, or even participating in sexual coitus or other forms of sexual contact unthink-able. Monroe E. Greenberger, M.D., a urologist affiliated with New York University Medical School, cited pelvic discomfort, a burning feel-ing in the penis during urination and after ejaculation, and hematosper-mia (slight bleeding during ejaculation) as possible problems associated with improper prostate function. Martin K. Gelbard, M.D., a urologic surgeon and clinical assistant professor of urology at the UCLA School of Medicine, says painful burning on ejaculation is also a sign of possi-ble inflammation of the prostate or a bacterial infection lurking within the gland.

The prostate gland, which is situated in a precarious spot (see Figure 1.2), is a major source of many problems related to male sexual health. As you can see, this gland actually wraps around the urethra. As men age, the prostate gland enlarges, thus tightening its grip or hold on the urethra. As a reminder, it is the urethra through which urine and ejacu-late pass. While the prostate gland has no direct biological bearing on sexual function, an enlarged prostate called benign prostate hyperplasia (BPH) can become a source of major frustration in relationship to sex-ual health.

---

**SPECIAL NOTE**

Disorders of the prostate gland can be life threatening if left untreated, depending on the degree of the problem. Prostate cancer kills thou-sands of men each year. Males of African descent, as a point of refer-ence, have a higher incidence of prostate cancer than any other nationality not only in the United States, but throughout the world.

Kent Wallner, M.D., a urologist who specializes in the treatment of prostate cancer at Memorial Sloan-Kettering Cancer Center in New York City, states that "prostate cancer is a very common disease and is more prevalent as men get older, with 15% of men at age 55 contracting can-cer, 30% by age 65 and the number skyrockets to 45% at age 75."

## Loss of Sexual Desire

In the introduction to Part II, I asked a number of questions, including "When was the last time you initiated sex with your partner?" If you have to think hard here, and your apparatus is still working, you for some reason have lost your sex drive. Loss of sexual desire is a universal problem, affecting both males and females, of all ages, nationalities, ethnic backgrounds, and socioeconomic levels. While the problem is usually associated with aging, current knowledge holds that many factors—including stress, alcohol, hormonal levels, fatigue, medications, insomnia, infections, traumatic experiences, repressed anger, and depression—can play a role in fading sexual desire. The list of possible causes of reduced libido is infinite and in itself requires a book-length discussion. Therefore, it is with this disorder that we find we have come full circle from the quote by Dr. Guirguis on the opening page of Part II.

Sue Johanson, R.N., the author of *Sex Is Perfectly Natural, but Not Naturally Perfect* (Penguin Books, 1991), tells us low sex drive is such a common problem that males and females suffer from it equally. Dr. Domeena Renshaw goes a step further, saying that lack of interest in sex is the second most common complaint patients have when making trips to their doctor's office.

As we have been stressing, sexual health is intimately linked to general health. According to Dr. William Regelson:

> Some feel that the essence of youth, indeed the essence of feeling fully alive—is libido. What I call the "youthful state" or the "youthful advantage" is, in reality, the ability to be stimulated and aroused by the environment that surrounds us. That is why I believe remaining sexually vital is often key to remaining youthful.

Medically, the evidence is mounting that this part of the human experience is as vital to long-term health as any other known biological, nutritional, or physiological factor that preserves life. And you play an important role in the preservation of this powerful force.

Despite the fact that the human male is physically capable of enjoying and experiencing a robust sex life indefinitely, it is not guaranteed. Many of the problems associated with men's sexual demise have complex origins, both of a physical and a psychological nature. On the other hand, lifestyle choices contribute to men's long-term sexual health more than previously thought. In addition, current data suggest that the aging male and inevitable sexual dysfunction are not one and the same.

In many respects loss of libido, loss of sexual desire, and erection problems can be characterized as silent or invisible illnesses: they are invisibly linked to your lifestyle habits and can take years to develop before becoming a chronic problem. In the next chapter, "The Forces Behind Sexual Dysfunction," we will take an in-depth look at this phenomenon.

# 6

# The Forces Behind Sexual Dysfunction

*The Best Prescription is Knowledge.*

C. Everett Koop, M.D.
*Former U.S. Surgeon General*

When our sexual prowess begins to falter, we tend to look outside of ourselves for the cause. Maintaining one's sexual health requires a lifetime commitment toward good health. Many of our sexual problems can be attributed to poor diet, lack of exercise, stress, pesticides, drugs, alcohol, or any of a number of other negative lifestyle factors. As stated above by Dr. Koop, "the best prescription is knowledge." I firmly believe that in the absence of congenital defects, a person who is experiencing sexual dysfunction is a person out of sync with the laws of nature.

What do we mean by "out of sync with the laws of nature"? More important, what are the laws of nature? "Out of sync" in this context simply refers to not following some basic laws or known principles that tend to naturally assist the body in its efforts to maintain health. Robert Willix Jr., M.D., a former open-heart surgeon in South Dakota who developed that state's first open-heart surgery program, now advocates prevention and appropriate lifestyle changes. This is echoed by Robin Landis, coauthor of *Herbal Defense* (Warner Books, 1997), who insists that nature has actually provided us with the tools to make the maintenance of health a simple task. She says:

> At the most basic level, health maintenance is relatively simple.
> Provide the body with a lot of what it needs; don't give it much
> of what it doesn't and the body will run itself.

We tend to disregard this fact, just as we disregard scientific evidence
at times. Emmanuel Cheraskin, M.D., William M. Ringsdorf, D.M.D.,
and J. W. Clark in the early 1960s reported their findings concerning
poor nutritional and lifestyle habits being a major cause of degenerative
diseases. Their research, presented in the highly acclaimed book *Diet
and Disease* (Keats Publishing, 1968), was met with fierce opposition
from the medical community.

Kurt Donsbach, D.C., Ph.D., N.D., director of the Hospital Santa
Monica in Rosarity Beach, Mexico, notes that for years even the prestigious National Cancer Institute insisted that there is no correlation between the development of cancer and one's dietary habits. Of course,
this is now known to be incorrect.

What has all this got to do with maintaining your sexual health? In
this chapter, we will look at why many sexual health and alternative
health professionals claim that, to some extent, you play a major role in
preserving your sexual potential. The fact is that your sexual health and
general health are one and the same. The list below presents but a small
sampling of the many forces that can destroy your sexual nature. For
the most part, these negative forces are a direct result of faulty lifestyle
habits or a disregard of the basic health maintenance laws defined by
Robin Landis.

## Alcohol, Caffeine, and Nicotine

It is common knowledge that smoking can cause cancer and that excessive alcohol consumption can cause cirrhosis of the liver. Not only can
these diseases ruin your sexual health, but they can compromise your
general health and shorten your life expectancy. People who rely on caffeine to meet the energy demands of their body put undue stress on their
adrenal glands. The adrenal glands play a role in the manufacture of sex
hormones as well as in helping our bodies adapt to stressful situations.
Individuals suffering from exhausted adrenal glands exhibit a marked
decrease in energy, as well as lethargy, dizziness, blood sugar disorders,
and food cravings.

Caffeine is not the only substance that negatively impacts adrenal function. Alcohol and nicotine do the same. These three substances have also been linked to disorders such as heart disease, kidney damage, and impaired nerve transmission. This is due in part to those agents' ability to constrict blood vessels, thus causing improper blood flow. Improper blood flow can cause high blood pressure, thus contributing to the vicious cycle and adding to the body's stress load plus inhibiting proper blood flow to the genitals.

## Arthritis and Degenerative Disorders

Disorders such as arthritis are usually associated with growing old. While arthritis and other degenerative disorders can strike at an early age, it is the pain and discomfort, not aging per se, that prohibit an enjoyable sexual experience. Chronic illness can dampen your lust and your sexual appetite.

## Chronic Fatigue

Sex, foreplay, and the emotional expenditure required to pursue and endure a sexual relationship demand energy—and lots of it. It is estimated that today Americans make more than 500 million office visits to doctors due to a general feeling of malaise and subtle feelings of fatigue. Many of these problems are attributed to improper lifestyle habits.

Individuals suffering from chronic fatigue syndrome (CFS), a severer form of unrelenting fatigue, often have to make drastic lifestyle changes to lead a normal life, not to mention to resume a healthy robust sex life.

## Diabetes

According to urologists Dr. David Mobley and Dr. Steven Wilson, 65 percent of males who develop diabetes become impotent within 10 years.

The problems associated with diabetes involve impaired circulation and nerve damage. Over time, diabetes causes contriction of the blood vessels. This causes the arteries to harden, further restricting blood flow.

This process is called arteriosclerosis. Diabetes also can cause nerve damage, called neuropathy, which prohibits proper nerve function. Many diabetic patients complain of numbness in their legs, hands, and feet.

Diabetic neuropathy and arteriosclerosis are major causes of impotency. They can also cause sexual problems for women. It is important to remember that strong and powerful erections depend on proper circulation, blood flow, and nerve transmission. Conversely, soft, pliable vaginal tissue and ample mucosal secretions in females also depend on these conditions.

## Elevated Cholesterol

About 5 percent of the individuals suffering from problems of a sexual nature can blame elevated cholesterol levels. When low-density lipoprotein (LDL) cholesterol levels are elevated, arteries can become clogged, impeding proper blood flow. For every 10 points above normal, according to Dr. Howard Peiper and Nina Anderson in *Natural Solutions for Sexual Dysfunction*, there is a 32 percent increase in a male's chance of becoming impotent. Elevated cholesterol levels are also a major risk factor of heart disease.

## Hypertension

Hypertension (high blood pressure) is a major cause of erectile dysfunction in males and impaired blood flow to the genitals in females. While many people associate these problems with the medications used to treat high blood pressure (which can also contribute to the problems), narrowing of the blood vessels is the underlying culprit. Erections are based on blood engorgement, as are sensory feelings in the female external sexual organs to some extent.

## Lack of Exercise

If regular exercise is not one of your lifestyle habits, you may be putting your sexual and general health in serious jeopardy. Exercise keeps your heart strong and increases its ability to pump blood, helping to supply blood and oxygen to organs and cellular structures. Lack of regular exercise promotes weight gain, slows down the elimination of waste byproducts, and contributes to weakened arteries and blood vessels. These can definitely put your sexual appetite on ice.

## Lack of Information

To maintain your health and your sexuality, you need to understand how your sexual system operates. Knowing how your body works can help you make adjustments to adapt to your changing sexual makeup throughout your life cycle.

## Medical Conditions

There are a host of physical problems such as urinary tract infections, vaginal infections, interstitial cystitis (inflammatory bladder infection), and yeast infections that can tax the healthiest sex drive. These conditions can cause itching, burning, and pain in the vulva area of many females.

While antibiotics are the normal treatment for many of these conditions, they can upset the natural intestinal flora, thus causing the condition to flare again. Consuming yogurt with live bacterial cultures like *Lactobacillus acidophilus* and *Lactobacillus bifidus,* or using these as dietary supplements, can greatly assist you in your efforts to maintain your sexual health.

## Medications

There are many prescription drugs in addition to antibiotics that can have a negative impact on sexual health. It is a well-known fact that drugs used to treat high blood pressure and depression can diminish the sex drive. Paradoxically, birth control pills, which alter the process of fertilization, can also decrease your interest in sex.

## Psychological Factors

It is well known that psychological factors such as stress, mental fatigue, depression, anxiety, panic attacks, lack of self-confidence, and relationship issues can diminish sexual desire, drive, and motivation. Resolving conflicts and other psychological issues is vital to restoring sexual libido, as evidenced by many of the sexual problems with psychological origins that we reviewed in Chapters 4 and 5. How interwoven is your state of mind with your sexual health? To fully grasp the degree of the mind-body connection, consider the following statement made by Paavo Airola, N.D., Ph.D., author of *How to Get Well* (Health Plus Publishers, 1989):

> If the patient is under a severe stress or acute anxiety, his or her ability to absorb and utilize nutritional and medicinal factors will be seriously impaired, and the expected healing will not manifest as long as the emotional disturbance continues to act.

We will discuss this in more detail in Chapter 15, "Sometimes You Just Have to Unplug." An early pioneer in the use of natural alternatives to treat disorders caused by unhealthy lifestyle choices, Dr. Airola believed that nonadherence to the biological laws that foster good health is the root cause of disease.

## Stress and Emotions

The process of disconnecting, according to Robert Hirschfield, M.D., chairman of the Department of Psychiatry and Behavioral Sciences at the University of Texas Medical Branch at Galveston, is rampant. Dr. Hirschfield insists that patients who experience sexual problems should not always blame their hormones or neurochemicals (brain chemicals such as dopamine). According to Dr. Hirschfield, "the most common cause of sexual problems is relationship issues, not medication and not depression." The stressors of everyday living can creep into a relationship and have devastating consequences sexually and emotionally.

We will cover this in more detail in Chapter 15.

## Thyroid Problems

The thyroid gland is located in your neck, below your voice box. It controls your metabolic process, which determines how fast your body converts food to fuel. Your thyroid helps regulate your weight, energy levels, body temperature, oxygen consumption, and tissue growth. It also helps keep you energetic; functions in the development of bone, nerves, and the reproductive organs; and helps fuel your sex drive. All this is accomplished by the release of the thyroid's most active hormones, $T_4$ and $T_3$. Thyroid-stimulating hormone (TSH) also plays a role in the gland's proper function.

In the absence of any physiological or congenital defects, the thyroid gland can be severely hampered in its metabolic actions by inactivity or lack of exercise. Consumption of processed, refined foods, as well as white flour and sugar, can suppress the dynamic actions of this small but powerful gland. Saturated fats, sugary soft drinks, alcohol, excessive salt, coffee, tea, and nicotine can all tax the thyroid.

To add to the problems, according to Phyllis A. Balch, C.N.C., and James F. Balch, M.D., authors of *Prescription for Nutritional Healing* (Avery, 2000), the drug levothyroxine (Synthroid) widely used to treat thyroid conditions can cause a 13 percent loss in bone mass. They estimate that at least 19 million people across the country are on this drug to treat improper thyroid function.

Michael Murray, N.D., author of *Dr. Murray's Total Body Tune-Up* (Bantam Books, 2000) has found in his research that improper thyroid function can cause depression and a loss of libido.

## Toxic Overload

It is a known fact that aging causes a shift in hormone production. However, scientists now know that the chemicals used to process our food, clean our water, and fertilize our soil, as well as the hormones given to many of the animals in our food supply, cause metabolic imbalances. From altering our DNA (our genetic blueprint) to affecting the transmission of messages by our hormonal system, today's environmental hazards are increasing the number of individuals who are sexually dysfunctional or sterile.

Sherry Rogers, M.D., who specializes in environmental medicine, reminds us that there are a massive number of chemicals and pesticides to which we are exposed today that didn't exist in years past. These foreign chemicals are called xenobiotics, according to Dr. Rogers. We have some inborn capabilities for metabolizing these substances and ridding our bodies of them. However, Dr. Rogers maintains that the process she refers to as xenobiotic detoxification is dependent on our genetic, or inherited, ability to cleanse ourselves of waste products.

The last piece to this puzzle is concerned with the length, duration, and negative attributes of the chemicals present.

Dr. Andrew Weil concurs with Dr. Rogers's assessments. Dr. Weil states that "toxic overload may be a significant cause of allergy, autoimmune disease, and a host of other degenerative disorders." He says that "the medical profession and the scientific research community have been a little remiss and very slow to react to these facts." In his estimation, toxic overload is one of the greatest threats to health and well-being, not only here in the United States but throughout the world.

How toxic overload directly affects your ability to fully enjoy your sexuality is covered in Chapter 11, "Detoxify to Satisfy."

In the absence of any congenital defects, we can expect to enjoy and maintain our sexual health throughout our lifetime. For the most part, nature does decrease our production of hormones and other chemicals, which may cause us to react a little slower to sexual stimuli. Nonetheless, we have the ability to remain sexually active and vibrant under some extenuating circumstances. The farther removed we become from the basic laws of nature, the more we compromise our long-term sexual potential. The forces behind sexual dysfunction are infinite and ongoing. You can assist nature now in preserving your natural born sexuality by "living well." Or, you can disregard nature's basic laws and pay with the possible loss of your sexual capabilities and self-esteem. The forces behind sexual difficulties are in many cases a direct result of poor lifestyle habits.

In the next part, "Conventional Wisdom," we will explore the world of sex machines, drugs, and medical devices used to replace your natural ability to engage in sexual intercourse and boost the natural sensory abilities that enable you to enjoy the physical pleasures of human sexual contact.

# PART III

# CONVENTIONAL
# WISDOM

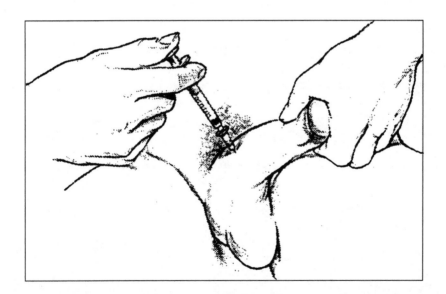

**FIGURE III.1.**They say a picture is worth a thousand words. How many words come to mind when viewing this illustration of a man giving himself a penile injection?

**Source:** David F. Mobley and Steven K. Wilson, *Reversing Impotence Forever!*, (Alvin, TX: Swan Publishing, 1995), p. 81.

Penile injection is one of the most popular methods of treating impotency. As shown in Figure III.1, it requires the user to inject a prescribed drug into his penile arteries. Although a very popular method, it has many drawbacks and complications, as I'm sure you've imagined.

For females suffering from inhibited arousal disorder, the Food and Drug Administration (FDA) recently approved the Eros-CTD, which is a device that fits over the clitoris. By pump activation it emulates manual or oral stimulation, and is highly erotic and titillating.

In Part III, we will look at some of the more popular devices, drugs, and other conventional protocols used to compensate for the loss of one's sexual capabilities.

The ability to give and receive love as expressed via sexual means is one of the most basic attributes we have as humans. Some people feel that maintaining it is as important as preserving life itself. This is evident by the extreme measures we as a species will take to participate in this three-letter act called sex.

Conventional wisdom focuses on the loss of sexual capabilities. You, however, should not. Preservation, enhancement, and development of your natural capabilities should be your focus. Conventional wisdom, however widespread it may be, is not the only alternative you have for preserving and enjoying your sexual potential.

# 7

*✑*

# Treatments and Devices

*For those with sex problems, a wider array of effective treatments is now available than at any previous time in history. The sex therapy introduced by behavior therapists Masters and Johnson in the 1960s and early 1970s has proved its worth, and there are also new and beneficial mechanical and medical methods.*

> Bernie Zilbergeld, Ph.D.
> *Codirector of Clinical Training,*
> *Human Sexuality Program,*
> *University of California at San Francisco*

As early as 1845, patent requests for inventions that related to sexual function, contraception, and desire were being submitted to the U.S. Patent Office. The first device given a patent was called the "wife protector," and was developed by Dr. John Beer in 1846. The device was a diaphragm fashioned after the small mirrors that dentists use to view the teeth. The device was the first that sought to give women some control over their sexuality as well as control birth, without interrupting orgasm. The small device was inserted into the vagina and was intended to prevent semen from reaching the uterus.

In 1988 a new era of implants began as technology advanced. As cited by Hoag Levins, author of *American Sex Machines* (Adams Media, 1996), many of the early surgical endeavors were frightening and almost Frankensteinist. He says that due to corporate backing and new technology, medicine began to shift its focus to direct surgical interventions and the interior of the penis. The goal was to build in practical terms a true bionic penis. Not to be outdone in the latter part of the nineteenth century, women saw patents for the first artificial breast submitted to the U.S. Patent Office. These artificial breasts were used until 1991, when researchers at the FDA confirmed that the polyurethane foam coverings in the implants broke down upon contact with human tissue. The foam actually transformed into a chemical called 2-toluene diamine (TDA). TDA, known to cause cancer in laboratory animals, is considered a hazardous waste product by the FDA.

We, as a species, are beginning to find more and more ways to extend our life span. But as Walter Pierpaoli, M.D., Ph.D, director of the Biancalana-Masera Foundation for the Aged in Ancona, Italy, says:

> What is tragic is to lose the physical strength and vigor that enables us to share life's pleasures. It is not enough to extend life unless we can also extend our ability and our desire to enjoy it and to relish the very things that make us happy to be alive.

In this chapter, we will review the conventional treatments and devices that men and women have used to improve their sexual functioning.

## The Male Options

Estimates indicate that only 5 to 10 percent of men seek medical help for problems related to impotency. Health officials expect that within the next few years the roughly 20 million American men who suffer from erectile dysfunction alone will increase to more than 47 million, according to Dr. Bernie Zilbergeld. This prediction is echoed by Tom F. Lue, M.D., a professor in the Department of Urology at the University of California in San Francisco who also serves as co-chairman of the Sexual Function Health Council of the American Foundation for Urologic Disease. According to Dr. Lue, the past decade has seen a variety of new treatment options ranging from penile implants, to vacuum devices, to new noninvasive drug therapies. The options, says Dr. Lue, enable physicians to now successfully treat impotency and other sexually related problems.

An additional problem in this scenerio is that when the projections become a reality and the number of dysfunctional men reaches the 47 million mark, it will also mean dysfunction for the men's 47 million partners. Furthermore, many men do not seek professional help due to embarrassment or a lack of knowledge concerning their treatment options. There are, however, a number of medical options available. Penile injection therapy, vacuum constriction devices, and penile prosthetic implants are the three major options used in the United States to treat more than 90 percent of all impotency cases.

## Penile Injection Therapy

As mentioned in the introduction to Part III, erection injections are one of the most popular methods employed by urologists to help males regain their ability to have erections sufficient enough to engage in sexual intercourse. The men, like diabetic patients who require insulin, are taught how to inject themselves with a small amount of medication, in this case directly into the corpora cavernosa of their penis. As you may have guessed, many men eventually have problems with maintaining this protocol. In fact, reports from as early as 1993 by the National Institutes of Health (NIH) cite the dropout rate to be extremely high. Officials claim that many men stop the treatment right after starting it.

Once an injection is given, it takes about 10 to 15 minutes for an erection to occur. The erections usually last for about 30 to 90 minutes. The procedure was first introduced in the United States by Dr. Giles Brindley, a neurophysiologist from Great Britain. In 1982, at the American Urological Association's annual meeting in Las Vegas, Dr. Bindley actually injected himself to clarify his point. To the amazement of a stunned audience of his peers, Dr. Brindley lowered his pants and proclaimed that he had injected himself a few minutes before his presentation to show how relaxation of the muscles in the corpora cavernosa was responsible for allowing increased blood flow in the penile arteries, thus facilitating a normal erection. Dr. Mobley and Dr. Wilson state that this procedure "is effective in about 65% of the individuals who use it." They also mention that this protocol is very useful in treating impotency that is a result of spinal cord injuries.

One of the earliest drugs developed to facilitate blood flow to depressed arteries was phentolamine. According to Dr. Mobley and Dr. Wilson, it was combined with the drug papaverine to enhance its action.

However, over time the combination of the two drugs presents some very disturbing complications. For example, the drugs can cause:

- Priapism to develop. Priapism, or prolonged erection, is a serious condition and warrants medical attention. Left untreated, priapism can cause permanent erectile dysfunction.
- Bruising of the penile tissue due to the repeated injections.
- Extensive formation of scar tissue.
- Resistance to the medication. Eventually even high dosages will not result in an erection.
- Pain at the site of the injections.

By 1994, papaverine had fallen from favor with many urologists in the United States due to the fear of lawsuits. Today, it is available only from foreign manufacturers, which further clouds the issue of its safety and effectiveness.

## Vacuum Constriction Device

The vacuum constriction device, also known as the pump, can be compared somewhat to the air pumps used to inflate tires. However, the apparatus is placed over the penis and the air is removed from the cylinder-like device, using a manual or electric pump. (See Figure 7.1.) This causes an erection by forcing blood into the erectile tissue. The blood is then trapped by tightening an elastic band called a constriction ring around the bottom of the penile shaft.

Clients who use a vacuum constriction device tend to stop within one year after starting. The extended time it takes to obtain a erection, the loss of foreplay, and intimacy issues can affect a couple's attempts to bond. Frustration over unsuccessful attempts to reach ejaculation due to the penile constriction ring at the base of the penis also can present problems. The overriding positive of this treatment is that it is noninvasive. The patient can see through the plastic chamber as the negative pressure draws the blood into his penis. At that point he or his partner can place the constriction ring around the penis.

Richard Milsten, M.D., director of the Center for Sexual Health in Woodbury, New Jersey, and Julian Slowinski, a senior clinical psychologist at Pennsylvania Hospital in Philadelphia and a certified sex therapist, insist that the constriction ring shouldn't be left in place for longer than 30 minutes.

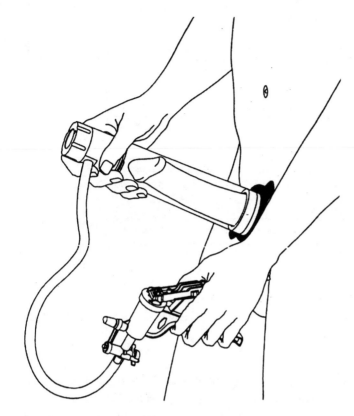

**FIGURE 7.1.** A vacuum constriction device.

Source: David F. Mobley and Steven K. Wilson, *Reversing Impotence Forever!* (Alvin, TX: Swan Publishing, 1995), p. 79.

## Penile Prosthetic Implants

A prosthesis is defined as an artificial part to replace a natural part of the body. Penile prostheses are actually surgically implanted into the penis. The first U.S. patent for a semirigid instrument to be surgically implanted into the penis for the purpose of causing erections was awarded on September 3, 1974. It was given to Viktor Konstantinovich Kalnberz of the Soviet Union for a device called the Bionic Penis. (See Figure 7.2.) Kalnberz's philosophy concerning the use of this type of device was the fact that it was concealed and had several psychological advantages.

In 1984 Dr. Tom Lue and colleagues at the University of California

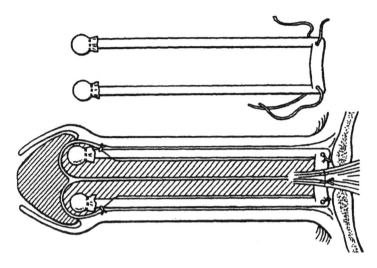

**FIGURE 7.2.** Viktor Kalnberz's Bionic Penis.

**Source:** Hoag Levins, *American Sex Machines* (Holbrook, MA: Adams Media, 1996), p. 133.

invented the penile pacemaker, which they fashioned after the heart pacemaker. Tiny electronic devices known as electrodes are surgically inserted around the nerves near the prostate gland. These are the nerves that when stimulated have a profound effect on penile erections. To initiate an impulse, a man presses a button on an instrument about the size of a garage door opener.

---

**SPECIAL NOTE**

Removal of the prostate gland due to cancer can render many men impotent. Dr. Patrick Walsh of Johns Hopkins has devised a procedure that focuses on preserving the integrity of the nerve fibers near the prostate gland that initiate erections. While this nerve-sparing procedure has seen great success rates, it is not 100 percent failure-proof.

---

Another type of penile prosthesis is the inflatable or hydraulic prosthesis. This type of prosthesis is placed in the penis through a surgical incision made in either the scrotum or the abdomen. Two balloon-like cylinders that are designed to expand are put into the corpora cavernosa. A button-like apparatus is pressed to stimulate or to stop an erection. Some common drawbacks associated with this type of penile implant include:

- Fear of injury during sexual intercourse.
- Cost of the procedure and possible insurance company regulations concerning paying for it.
- Potential surgical complications.
- Possible breakage or fracture of the prosthesis during sexual intercourse.
- Mechanical failure of the device.
- Damage to any functional erectile tissue during implantation of the prosthesis.
- Erosion of the device through the skin over time.
- Psychological issues.

All of the procedures, thus far discussed require an adjustment in thinking. Both partners must accept and adjust to this part of their sexuality. Peter Kilmann, Ph.D., and Katherine H. Mills, Ph.D., authors of *All About Sex Therapy* (Plenum Press, 1983), state that "a partner who is not in favor of the prosthesis likely will not help the man's adjustment to it."

## Other Male Options

It is important to remember that one size often does not fit all. Medical doctors will also suggest surgery to increase blood flow to the penile arteries. Revision surgery may be necessary in some cases, as devices like the inflatable prosthesis may not last a lifetime. Surgery to repair what is known as venous leakage is also sometimes necessary. Venous leakage in recent years has come to be thought of as much more of a problem than previously realized in relation to impaired blood flow to the penile arteries. The goal of surgery here is to correct imperfections in the erectile tissue that cause it to no longer act like suction cups, forcing blood into the penis, and then via that suction forcing the veins in the penis that urologists call emissary veins to hold the blood in. In venous leakage, blood may enter the erectile chambers, but it leaks out, thus preventing the man from maintaining an erection.

In addition to surgery, the other male options include drugs, hormone replacement therapy, M.U.S.E., and $PGE_1$.

### Drugs

Viagra and other drugs are now widely used to treat male impotency. Viagra will be covered in more detail in the next chapter.

### Hormone Replacement Therapy

New evidence indicates that men actually suffer from what doctors call male viropause. Similar to women in menopause, men in viropause can try hormone replacement therapy (HRT), mainly testosterone, to offset the effects of aging on sexuality. This is done via testosterone patches, injections, and other delivery systems.

HRT is controversial and not recommended by many physicians unless blood tests show reduced blood levels. Testosterone is what actually fuels prostate-related cancers.

### Medicated Urethral System for Erections

The medicated urethral system for erections is more commonly known as M.U.S.E. The procedure involves injecting a dissolvable pellet into the urethra prior to intercourse. Erection generally occurs within 10 minutes.

### Prostaglandin E$_1$

Prostaglandin E$_1$ (PGE$_1$) is a hormone-like substance approved for use in the United States in the 1990s. It is injected into the penis to produce an erection. However, it is expensive and has a short shelf life (6 months even when refrigerated). In addition, it doesn't work as well as when it is combined with papaverine and phentolamine, according to Dr. Mobley and Dr. Wilson.

## The Female Options

Just like men, women encounter many problems associated with sexuality. However, as we learned in Chapter 4, female sexual disorders were for many decades labeled as all-in-your-head conditions. In more scientific terms, problems of a sexual nature were for women classified as being psychological or emotional in origin. Take, for example, a prolapsed (fallen) uterus. During the eighteenth and nineteenth centuries, this disorder was not discussed by medical professionals because female private parts (genitals) were considered to be unmentionable. This practice was so endemic that medical students at the time were taught to make decisions regarding women's sexual and gynecological needs without even visually examining their genitals.

This was the dark age in regard to treatment options for women's sexual health issues as well as overall health issues. This era was also marked by very little data concerning women's health available to either medical personnel or laypersons.

Medically, during the early part of the twentieth century, the field of human sexuality began to open. This was accompanied by the introduction of an abundance of inventions that addressed women's sexual needs. The first electric-powered vibrational vaginal probe was introduced in 1911. Other inventions were aimed at clitoral stimulation such as an instrument called the "device for promoting marital accord." Since 1930 there has been an explosion of so-called sex toys designed to heighten female sexual response. For the first time, couples were encouraged to discuss sexual problems and seek out professional help to correct them.

The field of female sexuality, in many experts' opinion, is still in its infancy. Health professionals consider the body of knowledge concerning women's sexual issues lacking when compared to that for males. This situation was underscored by a report in the *Journal of the American Medical Association* in 1999. The study focused on the prevalence of sexual disorders in the United States. The investigators found that 43 percent of American women, both young and old, suffered to a greater degree from problems related to sexual health than did men. Only 31 percent of the males in this report had any problems concerning sexuality.

This belief that more women than men suffer from sexual problems is really mistaken, since I have found that the prevailing mind-set is that males suffer to a greater degree from problems related to sexual decline. This fallacy, however, has brought an array of treatment options to women suffering from inhibited sexual arousal and loss of sexual desire. Dr. Jennifer Berman is one of a very small number of female urologists who specialize in issues affecting female sexuality. She believes women can benefit from the same medical considerations given men. Dr. Berman says that "medical science is still perhaps a half-century behind in reference to the female pelvic anatomy." She insists that less is known about female pelvic anatomy than was known 30 years ago about male genital anatomy. Women do now have a number of medical options. We will review these in the remainder of this chapter.

## Clitoral Stimulation Device

In 2000, the FDA gave clearance for the marketing of a device called the EROS clitoral therapy device. Made by UroMetrics, Inc, a firm located in St. Paul, Minnesota, the instrument can only be prescribed by a physician. It is the first FDA-approved mechanism to treat female sexual arousal disorders. The device includes a small vacuum cup that is placed over the clitoris just before sexual intercourse or a sexual encounter. A vacuum pump that is about the size of the palm of your hand draws blood into the clitoris using suction. The purpose of the device is to increase blood flow to the clitoris to heighten sexual arousal. The clitoris is the female organ whose major function is to increase female sexual desire.

To find out more about this device, contact the Office of Public Affairs of the Food and Drug Administration at 1-800-INFOFDA. You can also find information on the web at http://www.fda.gov/bbs/topics/answers/anjo1012.htm/.

## Dilators

Dilators are used to treat the complications associated with vaginismus. These devices are used by sex therapists to help female clients retrain their vaginal muscles to accept penile penetration. Patients and their partners are instructed to use various-size dilators during foreplay sessions.

## Drugs

Viagra for women? Yes, this is a possibility in the very near future. Scientists believe that Viagra can help women the same way it does men: by increasing the blood flow to the genital area, thus improving the response to sexual stimuli. Although currently, Viagra has not yet been approved to treat sexual dysfunction in women, preliminary trials have shown some positive results. In some cases, however, Viagra has not shown any improvement in sexual response, according to Dr. Steven Kaplan at the Columbia Presbyterian Center in New York.

Other drugs are also often used to treat sexual problems in women. They include the following.

### Tranquilizers
Tranquilizers are used to help women with vaginismus to relax. This is to help the women be more receptive to sexual intercourse. Masters and

Johnson consider this approach illogical. In their opinion, this treatment doesn't take into consideration possible anatomical abnormalities or problems with self-esteem, body image, or relationship issues.

### Phentolamine, Apomorphine, Levodopa

According to Dr. Judith Reichman, phentolamine and apomorphine, drugs used to treat male impotency, provide similar benefits to women. Phentolamine increases blood flow by dilating the blood vessels, while apomorphine stimulates the central nervous system.

Levodopa, more commonly known as L-dopa, is well known for its use in combating the negative aspects of Parkinson's disease. L-dopa blocks the release of prolactin. As discussed in Chapter 2, prolactin is a hormone that decreases the sex drive. L-dopa causes an increase in the production of the brain neurotransmitter dopamine. As you know, dopamine is a highly stimulative sexual chemical. L-dopa, like most drugs, has a number of problematic side effects, such as headaches, vomiting, heartbeat irregularities, and nausea.

### Buproprion

A popular drug used to treat heart disease, buproprion offsets the negative side effects that antidepressant drugs have on the libido. Researchers are starting to look at its use by individuals not taking an antidepressant.

## Hormone Replacement Therapy

For women reaching menopause, healthcare professionals recommend hormone replacement therapy to offset the problems of sexual decline that are associated with menopause. The hormones estrogen and progestin are mainly used. Progestin is the synthetic version of progesterone. Physicians know now that using estrogen alone can increase problems with the endometrial lining of the uterus. Rapid and uncontrolled growth can occur, and is associated with increased risk of endometrial cancer.

## Testosterone

As already discussed, sexual health advocates insist that estrogen replacement is only part of the picture in relation to sexual health. To fully restore lost libido, they believe that androgen replacement is even more important. For women, the primary androgen with which to supplement is testosterone.

## Estradiol Vaginal Ring

Estrodiol is the most potent form of the three types of estrogen naturally produced by women. Estradiol vaginal rings, also known as estrings, are placed in the vagina like a diaphragm and gradually release small amounts of estrogen to the vaginal tissue. The purpose of the treatment is to fight vaginal atrophy.

## Vagifem

Vagifem is similar to the M.U.S.E. system for men. Instead of injecting a small pellet into the urethra, female patients put a small tablet into their vagina once daily for two weeks, then twice weekly. The purpose is to deliver estrogen to the vaginal tissue to restore lubrication, stimulate nerve endings, and decrease irritation and other symptoms of hormonal decline.

## Hormonal Creams

Many sexual health officials recommend using estrogen and testosterone creams to increase lubrication in the vagina. The creams are applied directly to the inside of the vagina, the inner labia lips, and the clitoris. They have shown the ability to increase arousal in some women. In addition, they can rejuvenate thin vaginal tissue, thus decreasing the pain and irritation associated with vaginal tissue that has atrophied.

Presently more than 41 million women suffer from female sexual arousal disorder. These creams help increase blood flow and lubricating secretions, and are much more erotic and psychologically appealing than taking oral forms of hormones.

## Prostaglandin E$_1$ Cream

Like prostaglandin injections formulated for male impotency, prostaglandin E$_1$ cream is designed to heighten sexual arousal and orgasm. It is used in cases of vaginismus and female sexual arousal disorder.

## Lifestyle Counseling

While sex therapy is a great tool and serves as a cornerstone in treatment, lifestyle counseling is becoming more commonplace. According to the health Website www.drkoop.com, "Impairment in sexual functioning can occur over time affecting different stages of the sexual response cycle." The following lifestyle problems are cited as causes and risk factors of sexual decline:

- Adrenal disorders
- Alcohol
- Chronic fatigue
- Circulatory problems
- Depression
- Diabetes neuropathy
- Drug abuse
- Emotional factors
- Guilt
- Interpersonal problems
- Lack of sexual activity
- Lack of trust
- Obesity
- Sexual fears
- Smoking
- Stimulants

## Perinometer

A perinometer, while not directly used to stimulate sexual desire, can measure the strength of your vaginal muscles. With this knowledge you can increase your awareness of your muscles, facilitating better control and relaxation during sexual intercourse. This can be of great benefit when treating vaginismus.

## Psychological Evaluation

One of the cornerstones of effective sex therapy is psychological counseling. Improving communication skills, uncovering deep-seated emotional trauma, and working on relationship issues are vital and in many cases are the foundation to restoring sexual zest and zeal.

You do not have to become a victim to poor sexual health. It is never too late to start a rejuvenation plan. Your body has some very powerful capabilities, especially when given the right tools, as well as an innate capability to repair and defend itself simultaneously. Many of the medical options discussed in this chapter can be a valuable part of your rejuvenation plan. In the next chapter, however, we will discuss why some medical options can be dangerous.

# 8

# Dying to Have Sex

*In the continuous quest for sexual exciters, enablers and enhancers drugs have been a constant wishful possibility despite the fact that many have been dangerous and most of them ineffective with often seriously dangerous side effects.*

Raymond L. McIlvenna, Ph.D.
*The Pleasure Quest: The Search
for Aphrodisiacs* (The Institute for Advanced
Study of Human Sexuality, 1988)

Thomas Edison once said that the doctor of the future will not give his or her patients any harmful drugs, but instead will interest them in the care of the human body via diet, and in the cause and prevention of disease. This, however, has not yet come to pass for our present society. According to recent reports, at least two-thirds of the American population use some type of prescription drug. Current estimates show that 75 million Americans are taking one or more drugs on a regular basis. The number of prescriptions written in this country per year has now reached 3 billion. This figure is almost double the number of ten years ago and is expected to double again in the new millennium.

Among the drugs used by Americans are drugs intended to alleviate sexual problems and enhance sexual performance. In this chapter, we will discuss how some of these drugs have serious side effects, which for some drugs include death.

# The Intended Action of Drugs

A drug is defined as a chemical substance taken to cure disease or improve health. According to the *Nursing 2002 Drug Handbook* (Springhouse Publishing, 2001), administration of any drug provokes a series of physiochemical events within the body. The first thing that occurs when a drug is taken is that it is absorbed at different sites on the cells called receptors. This is known as drug action. The second thing that happens is that the drug interacts with the body and exhibits its attributes. This is referred to as drug effectiveness.

James W. Long, M.D., who served on the faculty of the George Washington University School of Medicine for more than 35 years, maintains that most drugs are chemicals that are alien to the natural body chemistry. He says that "when a patient takes any prescribed drug for the first time there is always an inescapable element of uncertainty." According to Dr. Long, the reasons for this are crystal clear.

The first reason is related to the chemical nature of the drug. No drug exhibits a single action. Because of the complex nature of body chemistry, for a drug to be effective, it must be active enough to alter the body chemistry to a considerable degree. Additionally, it is virtually impossible to make a drug that will restrict its actions to a single area or body part. Hence the alteration of unintended metabolic processes, resulting in unwanted side effects and reactions.

The second reason is related to the unpredictability of patient responses to medication. Since no two people are alike, not all people will respond the same way to a medication.

These beliefs also are expressed in *The Patient's Desk Reference* (Macmillan, 1994). The authors of this drug reference book, Melvyn N. Freed and Karen J. Graves, maintain that although all drugs are tested exhaustively before being released into the marketplace, their absolute safety can never be guaranteed. In fact, these authors point out that it is common for a drug to pass all its clinical trials, then exhibit a rare toxic effect for the first time when thousands of people are taking it.

This statement has been proven accurate lately, as eleven major prescription drugs have been recalled in the last 4 years. These recalls have caused great concern, since only eight prescription drugs had been removed from the marketplace in the last 25 years before that. The drugs were removed from the marketplace because they either seriously injured or killed thousands of patients. In June 1998, according to the *Wall*

*Street Journal,* the maker of the sex drug Viagra reported sixteen deaths to the FDA.

Also, in a study reported in *The Lancet,* investigators found that between 1983 and 1993 there was a 150 percent increase in the number of deaths among outpatients who used prescription drugs. In addition, the authors concluded that outpatients were six times more likely to die as a result of mismanagement or overdose of prescribed medication in the United States.

Daniel Hussar, a professor of pharmacy at the Philadelphia College of Pharmacy, believes that this problem will continue to escalate. Andrea Knox, in her exposé "New Drugs Bringing More Risk and Recalls," published in the *Philadelphia Enquirer* in 2001, cites poor monitoring, speedy drug approvals, and aggressive advertising as major causes for the mounting problems associated with prescription drugs. In a commentary, "Time to Act on Drug Safety," published in the *Journal of the American Medical Association* in 1998, a note was made of the fact that the FDA has more than 1,400 staff members, but that only 52 people are actually responsible for overseeing the safety of the up to 5,000 brand name, generic, and over-the-counter drugs that are currently on the market. The remaining 1,300-plus staff members are responsible for approving new drugs. According to many health officials, this current situation is a cause for great concern. Professor Hussar suggests that eventually the American people will say that enough is enough.

Recognizing that this problem has reached epidemic proportions, the president's budget slotted $1.414 billion for the Food and Drug Administration in fiscal year 2002. This represented an increase of $123 million, or 9.5 percent, over the amount designated in fiscal year 2001. According to the *FDA Backgrounder,* an FDA consumer publication spotlighting health frauds, $10 million of the budget amount was to be used to protect patients against the negative aspects of prescription drugs, biological agents, and medical devices. It was the FDA's hope that it would be able to set up programs to better monitor drugs and other medical products on the market.

The sad facts according to recent data are that:

- More than one million people are accidentally injured every year in the United States as a result of medical therapy.
- More than 98,000 deaths occur due to preventable medical errors.

- Adverse drug reactions account for more than 2,216,000 serious side effects and more than 106,000 deaths in the United States.

To learn about the FDA's budget, go to http://www.fda.gov/opacom/backgrounders/budget.html. To find out more about drug recalls by the FDA, go to medwatch@listmanager.fda.gov.

## Viagra—Death by Normal Ingestion

It is apparent that you may be putting your long-term health in jeopardy by using drugs like Viagra to help meet your sexual needs. There have been several deaths linked to this popular drug used to treat impotency. Studies conducted at Cedars-Sinai Medical Center in Los Angeles found a direct link to a standard dose of Viagra. Sanjay Kaul, M.D., cited the results of data collected on 1,473 adverse reactions to Viagra, at the American College of Cardiologists' recent meeting in Anaheim, California. Dr. Kaul reported that 522 people had died, with more than 70 percent of those deaths occurring in men who had taken a standard dose of 50 milligrams of Viagra. The most frightening aspect of the report was that the majority of the deaths occurred in men under 65 years of age who had had no prior cardiac problems. To find out more about this study, go to http://www.sciencedaily. com/release/2000/03/0034031715.html.

Researchers now know there is an increased risk for individuals suffering from cardiovascular disease who use nitrates, which are found in nitroglycerine tablets. Nitrates are placed under the tongue to relieve angina (chest pain) due to heart disease. The brand-name nitrates currently prescribed include:

- Cardilate
- Iso-Bid
- Nitro-Bid (ointment)
- Nitrocid
- Nitro-disc
- Nitrogard (skin patches)
- Nitroglyn
- Sorbitrate (chewable tablets)

The reason nitrates and Viagra don't mix is that nitrates, like Viagra, can cause the blood pressure to drop. When the two drugs are combined, they can cause the blood pressure to plummet to seriously low levels. When this happens, the body tries to compensate by boosting the heart rate, which can lead to cardiac arrest. Current data show that at least two-thirds of the deaths linked to Viagra occur within 4 to 5 hours after ingestion of the medication.

In the Cedars-Sinai study, of the ninety patients who were using nitrates, 68 percent died, while 88 percent of those who died did so due to myocardial infarction (heart attack). Many of the individuals who died had never used nitrates. Murray A. Mittleman, M.D., and physicians at Beth Israel Deaconess Medical Center in Boston contend that many males who suffer from impotency have heart problems and other risk factors for heart disease. Based on his analysis of data on more than 4,000 men who took Viagra and more than 3,000 men who took placebo (a substance with no medical or nutritional value), Dr. Mittleman concluded that many of them, if they died, would probably die of a heart attack anyway due to their other risk factors.

In addition to death, Viagra has a number of other side effects, some serious, some just annoying. These other side effects include:

- Mild headaches
- Flushing
- Indigestion
- Runny nose
- Vision problems
- Chills
- Facial bloating
- Vomiting
- Gout attacks
- Abnormal electrocardiogram
- Anemia
- Hypoglycemia
- Blood sugar abnormalities
- Asthma
- Laryngitis
- Persistent cough
- Vertigo
- Unrealistic dreams
- Deafness
- Dry eyes
- Sleep disturbances
- Herpes simplex
- Urinary incontinence
- Ejaculation problems
- Bone pain
- Rectal bleeding

The problem most individuals have with Viagra is unrealistic expectations, according to Kenneth Brownstein, M.D., a clinical professor of urology at Thomas Jefferson University Hospital in Philadelphia, Pennsylvania. Many males, according to Dr. Brownstein, find that the drug does not correct erectile dysfunction. At least half of the individuals who use the drug find that it doesn't work for them, plus has side effects. Larry Katzenstein, a former medical editor of *American Health Magazine* and winner of the New York Newspaper Guild's Page One Award for Excellence in Journalism and the American College of Allergy and Immunology Media Award, cautions the general public in his book *Viagra: The Potency Promise* (St. Martin's Press, 1998) to "look before you leap." Mr. Katzenstein quotes Dr. Nachum M. Katlowitz, M.D., director of Male Sexual Function and Infertility at Maimonides Medical Center in Brooklyn, New York, as citing elevated levels of Viagra in the bloodstream of men taking the antibiotic erythromycin, the heartburn medication cimetidine (Tagamet), and the antifungal drugs ketoconazole and itraconzole. Researchers speculate that these, as well as other drugs, may elevate the blood levels of Viagra when the two are taken concurrently, suggesting that other drugs can interfere with the body's attempts to degrade (break down) and get rid of Viagra.

## Drugs Used to Treat Sexual Dysfunction

In addition to Viagra, a number of other drugs are commonly prescribed to treat sexual problems. Many of those sexual problems are side effects of the drugs used to treat depression, elevated cholesterol, menopausal symptoms, viropausal, high blood pressure, allergies, or anxiety disorders. These drugs for sexual problems include:

- Alprostadil
- Amantadine
- Apomorphine
- Betanechol
- Bromcriptine
- Buspirone
- Chlorpromaize
- Cyproheptaide
- Dipyridamole
- Estrogen
- Pentoxifulline
- Phentolamine
- Testosterone
- Thorazine
- Uprima
- Vasomax
- Vasotem
- Vassopression
- Verapamil
- Welbutrin

Taking all these drugs is not healthy. These drugs will only contribute to the toxic load your body has to handle. This can have long-term negative consequences on your liver function and on your body's ability to detoxify itself. In addition, all drugs have side effects, some mild, but some with long-term negative consequences. All these drugs are designed to treat symptoms, just like Viagra. They rarely correct the underlying cause of the problem.

As you can see, you may be compromising your sexuality simply by following your daily routine and taking your medications. There are literally hundreds of prescription and over-the-counter drugs that can contribute to sexual dysfunction. Do not, however, just stop taking any medication you may be using for medical reasons. On the contrary, discuss your situation with your healthcare professional and consider making some lifestyle changes that may benefit your efforts to regain your sexual vitality.

Henry I. Miller, M.D., a senior research fellow at the Hoover Institute and author of *Policy Controversy in Biotechnology* (Academic Press, 1997) reminds us that from 1990 to 1993, the average cost of bringing a single drug to the marketplace skyrocketed from $359 million to $500 million. Ironically, he notes, these drugs are still hazardous to your health and expensive to purchase. Dr. Miller served as an FDA official from 1979 to 1994.

Plato once said the direction of your education determines your future life. Learning about your medications may be one of the most important things you can do for your general health and your sexual potential. You don't have to be a victim of a for-profit society, as described by Dr. Mary Daly, Ph.D., quoted by Barbara Seaman and Gideon Seaman in *Women and the Crisis in Sex Hormones* (Rawson Associates, 1977), a book cited as one of the most important medical stories of the 1970s. Dr. Daly commented:

> We live in a society which is becoming one vast hospital. More and more individuals are being told that they and their children have been damaged by previous medication and that new treatment is required (because of) the consequences of the previous treatment.

In Part IV of this book, we will take an in-depth look at the natural alternatives at your disposal. Dr. Andrew Weil contends that many people are unaware of the existence of the natural, noninvasive healing systems throughout the world. This trend, however, is changing as evidenced by the recent results of *Prevention* magazine's annual International Wellness Study. This study is a global investigation into consumers' perceptions of and attitudes toward the healthcare arena.

The study revealed that more than 151 million Americans use natural supplements and herbal remedies daily. The survey also showed that 20.5 million consumers now opt to use herbal remedies in place of prescription drugs. This is because these people believe that living well is your best defense against illness and slowly developing degenerative conditions. Living well also is your best defense against many of the risk factors that are linked to sexual dysfunction. In Part IV, we will discuss how and why it is important to focus on prevention, rather than treatment, to regain and maintain your sexual vitality.

# PART IV

# THE NATURAL ALTERNATIVES

*There is a wonderful science in nature, in trees, herbs, roots, and flowers, which human kind has never yet fathomed. All the science and knowledge of our enlightened age, as taught in the colleges and universities, does not equal the science in nature, and yet that science is little understood even by the most intelligent people.*

Jethro Kloss
*Back to Eden* (Lotus Press, 1997)

Donald M. Vickery, M.D., former head of the Reston, Virginia Medical Center and the Community Medical Department of Georgetown School of Medicine, says in his book *Lifeplan for Your Health:*

> In this country (the United States) the emphasis for decades has been on research for cures rather than prevention. Little wonder we know a lot about treating these problems but not much about preventing them.

This emphasis Dr. Vickery mentions is changing rapidly. Many countries around the world have healthcare systems that are completely drugless. In many respects the United States is just beginning to catch up with the world. What we consider to be alternative treatments are in fact the primary form of healthcare in many of these countries. Over the last decade two landmark studies were conducted in the United States on the trend toward the preferential use of nonconventional healthcare modalities. These two studies, known together as the Eisenberg Report, were done in 1993 and 1998. The second study, published in the *Journal of the American Medical Association* on November 11, 1998, indicated that Americans had shifted gears and were looking for more noninvasive ways to maintain their health. They were placing more focus on prevention, and less focus on treatment via surgery or dangerous drugs. These reports showed that Americans were spending up to $13.7 billion on what are classified as nonmedical methods of treatment.

During the last several decades, the American public has been fighting to gain access to information on complementary treatment options, natural protocols, and nutritional supplements. As signed into law by President Bill Clinton, the Dietary Supplement Health and Education Act (DSHEA) of 1994 seeks to reduce Americans' ignorance concerning other healing systems, nutritional supplements, and natural programs. In response to public demand, Congress recently increased the budget of the NIH's National Center for Complementary Medicine from $50 million to $89 million. Additionally, the NIH's Office on Dietary Supplements had a $10 million budget in fiscal year 2002 to conduct research on the efficacy of herbs, amino acids, vitamins, minerals, and other items that are classified as dietary supplements.

In Part IV of this book, we will examine many of the nonconventional protocols, supplements, food programs, and other natural modalities that have been used to treat as well as prevent problems associated with sexual decline. Many of these modalities, some more than 5,000 years old, have now been proven effective by science. As nutritional researchers Dr. Emanuel Cheraskin and Dr. William Ringsdorf Jr., point out in their book *Psychodietetics,* "Any important 'new idea' has to go through three stages: first ridicule, then discussion, and finally, general acceptance.

While many healthcare professionals are still fighting the trend toward integrative medicine (which combines conventional and alternative medicine), nontraditional methods are becoming part of mainstream healthcare practice. Many nutritional supplements and natural protocols have a long history of safe and effective use for sexual concerns. Many effectively treat the underlying causes and not merely the associated symptoms. More important, they will not jeopardize your general health— or your sexual health—in the process.

# 9

# Proper Nutrition—Your Best Aphrodisiac

Every area concerning human sexuality has been intensively investigated, except the role of nutrition and how it affects a person's sex life. I have proven in countless cases that improper diet causes damage to and malfunction of the sex organs, and that prescribing an individual proper diet leads to restoration of the male's virility and the return of feeling to the female's genital area.

> Henry G. Bieler, M.D.
> *Dr. Bieler's Natural Way to Sexual Health* (Charles Publishing, 1972)

Biologically, it is evident from our discussion thus far that sexual vitality depends upon having adequate sex hormones, good sensory stimulation, and proper blood flow to the sexual organs and erectile tissue. Psychologically, a happy, active, stress-free person is much more likely to enjoy a long vibrant life filled with satisfying sexual encounters. Henry G. Bieler, M.D., an early pioneer of the medical application of clinical nutrition, felt that sexual dysfunction may have a nutritional origin. This belief, according to the late Paavo Airola, Ph.D., N.D., author of *Are You Confused?* (Health Plus Publishers, 1980), had originally been dismissed as sheer nonsense by modern science. However, Dr. Airola said:

There is a growing conviction among clinical nutritionists and some doctors that many sexual inadequacies and disorders, such as male impotency; female frigidity; male and female sterility; menstrual and menopausal disorders have nutritional origins.

Can food really increase your sex drive? Is it possible to restore male virility and sensory feeling to the female genitalia by nutritional means? Are you putting your sexual health in jeopardy through your diet? If you and your healthcare professional can't find a psychological or physiological reason for your diminishing sexual appetite, you may want to reexamine your current nutritional habits. Consider these facts alone:

- Consuming heavy meals can reduce male testosterone production by 50 percent.
- Inadequate water intake and chronic dehydration make it very difficult to maintain strong erections.
- A diet high in simple sugars can sap your energy and contribute to your low sex drive.
- A high-fat, low-fiber diet can clog your arteries, decreasing the blood flow to your sexual organs.
- Eating a high-protein meal with moderate carbohydrates can elevate your mood and increase your production of the brain chemicals that heighten sexual desire and sex drive.
- Without some fat and cholesterol in your diet, your body is unable to properly make the sex hormones.

In Chapter 9, we will explore the folklore and analyze the scientific data concerning nutrition and sexual health. We will learn how food affects your mood, alters your energy levels, and contributes to what health experts call nutritional diseases. It is in the area of nutrition that you can make the biggest difference in your sexual and overall health.

## Sex and Nutrition

The old adage that you are what you eat is accurate when it comes to sexual health. Health and longevity are rooted in proper nutrition. The human body is made up primarily of water. In fact, about 60 percent of the body is water. Also found in our tissues are proteins and various mineral elements. To rebuild all of its necessary components, the human body needs food. The entire human body including the sexual organs and sex hormones are made from food, air, and water. Dr. Airola maintained that nutrients are what the human body uses to reconstruct itself. He insisted that without a foundation of proper nutrition, all other modalities—including surgery, drugs, acupuncture, and chiropractic manipulation—will fail in the majority of cases. Elaine B. Feldman, M.D., professor of medicine and director of the Clinical Nutrition Research Unit at the Medical College of Georgia, states that "nutrition and exercise appear to be the two key elements in having a healthier middle and older age." She argues that these two areas are the building blocks, and to preserve your health in your later years, you must work on them in your younger years. Robert Sorge, N.D., Ph.D., director of the Abunda Life Health and Hotel Clinic in Asbury Park, New Jersey, reminds us that from a purely biological standpoint, no human is deficient in drugs, but 98 out of every 100 Americans are deficient in nutrients.

Morton Walker, D.P.M., author of *Sexual Nutrition* (Avery, 1993), contends that whole foods are what the doctors of the future will prescribe. He says that the thousands of biochemical and psychochemical processes that occur in a healthy body require the kind of nutrition only whole foods can provide. Whole foods are foods that have not been processed or refined.

## Fueling Your Sexual Organs

To fuel the sexual organs, help repair them, and maintain their function, Cynthia M. Watson M.D., author of *Love Potions* (Jeremy P. Tarcher, 1993) insists that at the very least, the body needs a diet rich in a variety of fresh fruits and vegetables, lean animal protein, and legumes. However, due to the highly processed nature of our current food supply, whole organic foods may be your best choice. The fresher the better.

### SPECIAL NOTE

Scientists today know that much of the soil in the United States is devoid of minerals and other vital nutrients. Therefore, it would be wise to incorporate a multiple-vitamin-and-mineral supplement into your daily dietary regimen.

Stephen Holt, M.D., FACP, president of the Illinois College of Physicians and Surgeons and author of *The Sexual Revolution* (Promotional Publishing, 1999), goes a step further. Dr. Holt reminds us that the ideal amounts of the nutrients required to maintain a sexually active and healthy individual are not readily available in the body. He says:

> In my own clinical experience, I have seen individuals reverse sexual problems by balancing their diet and taking well selected dietary supplements. Certainly they may have changed their lifestyle in other ways to enhance sexual function, but good nutrition is the foundation for continuing good sex.

When you view nutrition from this standpoint, it becomes evident that a proper diet is your most powerful aphrodisiac. What you eat affects not only your brain and how well it receives and transmits sexual stimuli, but also your entire hormonal system and the manufacture of your sex hormones. Eating a good diet could be compared to throwing more coal on a hot bed of flames. The key, however, is knowing how to manipulate this natural physiological mechanism. Barry Sears, Ph.D., in his landmark book *Enter the Zone* (Regan Books, 1995), puts this analogy into proper perspective:

> Food is far more important than just something you eat for pleasure or to appease hunger. It is a potent drug that you'll take at least three times a day for the rest of your life. Once food is broken down into its basic components (glucose, amino, and fatty acids) and sent into the bloodstream, it has a more powerful impact on your body and your health than any drug your doctor could ever prescribe.

Dr. Sherry Rogers tells us there is a nutrient that accomplishes the same function in the body as nearly every drug developed by man. Additionally Dr. Cynthia Watson reminds us of the sensual nature of food and of how we use food to entice our sexual partners and give it as gifts to promote sexual contact.

Food really can be a powerful aphrodisiac as well as your best medicine to keep those sexual flames burning now and in the future.

## Sex, Fat, and Cholesterol

One of the quickest ways to disrupt your natural hormonal balance is to go on an ultralow-fat diet. While we have been told to avoid fat because of its risk of causing hardening of the arteries, heart attacks, strokes, and elevated cholesterol levels, we need to consume some fat. It is true that saturated fats eaten in excess of your body's need can clog your arteries, impeding blood flow not only to your genitals, but also to your heart. This is something with which both males and females need to be

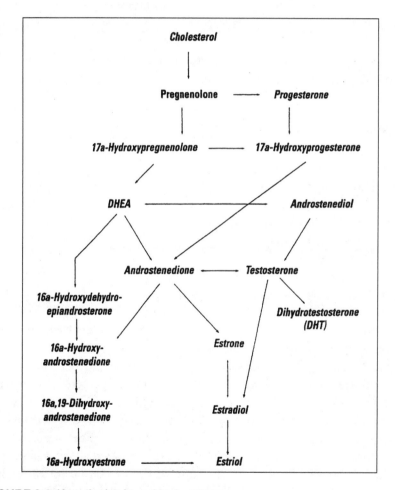

**FIGURE 9.1.** How the body makes hormones.

**Source:** Jonathan V. Wright and John Morgenthaler, *Natural Hormone Replacement* (Petaluma, CA: Smart Publications, 800-976-2783, 1997), p. 51.

concerned. At the same time, however, without enough cholesterol, the body is severely hampered in its efforts to make the steroid hormones, including estrogen and testosterone. As you can see in Figure 9.1, without cholesterol there is no starting point for the development of many of these small but powerful substances that fuel your sexual appetite.

It now becomes apparent that you need some fat in your diet. But how much? Presently there are a variety of opinions on the subject. Dean Ornish, M.D., recommends that no more than 20 percent of total calories be composed of fat. Other nutritional experts, such as Ann Louise Gittleman, author of *The 40/30/30 Phenomenon* (Contemporary Books, 1998), recommends a daily intake of up to 30 percent of calories from fat.

It is this author's opinion that the best diet is a moderate diet. The 40/30/30 dietary plan offers balance in nutritional terms, which promotes:

- Stabler blood sugar levels
- Stabler energy levels
- Better appetite control
- Better joint lubrication
- Better neurotransmitter activity
- Healthier skin and sexual organs
- Heightened sexual response
- Improved immune response
- Better nervous system and cell function
- Better moisture levels in the body organs

A 40/30/30 dietary regimen is composed of 40 percent carbohydrates, 30 percent protein, and 30 percent fat.

In addition to limiting your daily fat intake to 30 percent of your total calories, you should also get no more than 10 percent of your daily fat grams from saturated sources. Unsaturated and polyunsaturated fats should make up the bulk of your fat intake. Some unsaturated fats are actually good for you and essential for your health. They are called essential fatty acids for that reason. They are the fats that are responsible for helping the body accomplish many of the metabolic functions just listed. The essential fatty acids remain liquid at room temperature and include the omega-3s and the omega-6s.

However, while the unsaturated fatty acids in general have many health-building properties, the omega-6 fatty acids may contribute to high blood pressure, heart attacks, obesity, premature aging, and some forms of cancer. Some familiar sources of the omega-6 fatty acids are corn oil and borage oil. These fatty acids inhibit the aggregation of platelets and prevent blood clotting. These are risk factors that are certainly detrimental to sexual health. On the contrary, the omega-3 fatty acids such as flaxseed oil, walnut oil, and the fish oils (EPA and DHA) will assist you in your efforts to remain healthy and sexually active. There is mounting evidence that the omega-3 fish oils can reverse atherosclerosis, prevent heart attacks, reduce blood pressure, repair vascular deterioration, and keep the arterial walls pliable. All of these attributes, as we now know, are critical to maintaining good sexual health and to keeping your arteries free of unwanted cholesterol deposits.

But exactly what should you eat and what should you avoid? Reduce or eliminate the following:

- Bacon
- Cake
- Coconut oil
- Cured meats
- Doughnuts
- Egg yolks
- Fried foods
- Hot dogs
- Hydrogenated oils
- Ice cream
- Milk and dairy products
- Pork
- Potato chips
- Red meat
- Rich desserts
- Sausage
- White flour
- White rice
- White sugar

In place of the above-listed foods, consume the following:

- Brown rice
- Chicken and turkey
- Flax oil
- Raw fresh fruit
- Raw nuts
- Raw vegetables
- Soy meats and soy-based products
- Sherbet
- Vegetable oils like olive, canola, and peanut
- Whole-grain flour
- Whole grains
- Whole-grain cereals
- Yogurt

The bottom line: The omega-3s and other unsaturated fatty acids can decrease blood viscosity. In males, this will promote stronger penile erections. In females, it will promote proper blood flow to the external sexual organs, ensuring heightened sensory feeling and preservation of the vaginal tissue. The omega-3 and omega-6 fatty acids are important for preserving your sexual potential and overall health. To tip the scales in your favor, you should simply consume less of the omega-6s (but do not eliminate them) and more of the omega-3s.

## Sex, Food, and Mood

Can the food you ingest actually increase your sex drive? Can you with food reduce your stress and anxiety, and increase your potency, your vaginal secretions and lubrications, as well as your sensory feelings? The answer to all these questions is an astounding yes! Food is what provides the raw materials your body uses to manufacture your sex hormones. Contrary to popular belief, it is not a little blue pill prescribed by your doctor. Rather, by increasing the positive activity of your brain neurotransmitters, you can become highly stimulated, sexually motivated, and extremely aroused.

How can you do this? Easily, safely, effectively, and without the use of dangerous drugs such as antidepressants, narcotics, or alcohol (actually a central nervous system depressant). Neurotransmitters with the aid of various amino acids, vitamins, minerals, and other cofactors have a dynamic effect on your sexual thoughts, feelings, stamina, behavior (stress, anxiety, depression) and even sleeping patterns to some degree. By adjusting your food intake, you can increase your sexual performance twofold.

However, before we can master the ability to use our food intake to elevate our mood and sexual feelings, we need to know which brain chemicals we should manipulate. Following are nine key neurotransmitters, hormones, and amino acids:

- Acetylcholine. A neurotransmitter involved with memory, mental clarity, and concentration.
- Epinephrine. A highly stimulating hormone that helps the body ward off stress and keeps you energized.
- Norepinephrine. A hormone that is stimulating like epinephrine but to a lesser degree. It is the primary neurochemical used to fuel the sex drive.
- Dopamine. A neurotransmitter that stimulates alertness, excitement, and sexual desire.

- Growth-hormone-releasing factor. A hormone that directly affects your sexual drive, libido, passion, and sexual zest and zeal.
- Insulin. A hormone that assists the metabolism of carbohydrates by transporting them into the body cells.
- Serotonin. A neurotransmitter that promotes feelings of calmness, steadiness, and emotional tranquility.
- Tyrosine. An amino acid that elevates mood and functions in the production of dopamine and norepinephrine.
- Tryptophan. An amino acid that promotes sleep and relaxation.

Arthur Winter, M.D., and Ruth Winter, authors of *Eat Right, Be Bright* (St. Martin's Press, 1988), tell us that neurotransmitter-receptor interaction is directly influenced by what we eat and drink. But not only does what we eat affect the activity of neurotransmitters, it also determines how well they are manufactured. For example, many neurotransmitters are made from amino acids, the building blocks of protein, which we get from our diet. Other dietary substances, such as choline, a fatty substance sometimes classified as a vitamin, also play major roles in the manufacture of neurotransmitters. Judith Wurtman, Ph.D., a research scientist with the Massachusetts Institute of Technology (MIT), found that eating a meal composed predominantly of protein dramatically increases the production of dopamine and norepinephrine. Conversely, loading up on carbohydrates such as pasta and spaghetti will leave you feeling drained and lethargic due to elevated serotonin levels. Serotonin is made from the amino acid tryptophan, which promotes relaxation and sleep.

## The Carbohydrate Paradox

If you regularly indulge your sweet tooth or eat rich carbohydrate meals, you are slowly destroying your sexual potential. When you eat carbohydrates, you cause your body to produce insulin. Although insulin is responsible for transporting glucose (blood sugar) into the cells for energy, nutritionist Elizabeth Somer, author of *Food and Mood* (Henry Holt and Company, 1995), says it causes most of the amino acids circulating in the bloodstream to be absorbed into the body cells and not the brain cells. Tryptophan is the exception.

This is the carbohydrate paradox and the centerpiece of the sex-food-mood connection. Brian Morgan, Ph.D., and Roberta Morgan in their book *Brainfood* (H.P. Books, 1987), describe the brain's ability to let just selected nutrients into its tissues. This is known as the blood-brain barrier. Your brain needs a constant supply of glucose, which is provided by carbohydrates. Without a continuous level of 70 to 100 milligrams of glucose per 100 millileters of blood, your brain tunes out. Then you feel light-headed, dizzy, fatigued, confused, and just generally lethargic. However, if you sit down and have a rich carbohydrate meal, you will find yourself looking for the nearest sofa or chair. Not only will your sex drive go into the park position, but so will your mental clarity, stamina, and energy. This is caused by what health professionals call reactive hypoglycemia. That large carbohydrate meal you ate stimulated the hormone insulin. According to the Morgans, insulin causes the cells in the body to absorb the glucose from the blood, leaving little for the brain to use. Since glucose is our primary brain fuel, this leaves us in a state of confusion (brain fog), lifeless, and definitely not in a mind-set conducive to giving or receiving sexual pleasure. Additionally, most of the amino acids circulating in the bloodstream are absorbed into the body cells and not the brain cells. Consequently, the substances responsible for stimulating the brain chemicals that heighten sexual response, sex drive, and the levels of the sex hormones are short-changed.

The ideal thing to do is to balance your meals. Make sure you consume some protein (meat, chicken, fish, beans, lentils, shrimp, sunflower seeds, soy, eggs) with your carbohydrates. Eat in moderation and consume a variety of foods, including fresh fruits and vegetables. Remember that it takes protein about four hours to be properly digested and to kick in. By timing your food intake, as many professional and amateur athletes do, you will be ready, focused, highly motivated, and stimulated.

Consuming too much carbohydrates will not only contribute to the demise of your sexual energy, but may also cause impairment of your adrenal glands (where some of your sex hormones are made) and may eventually manifest itself as diabetes. It may also cause hardening of the arteries due to excessive storage of unwanted fat. This, as we know, can severely affect sexual potency.

## Sex and Other Food Culprits

By now you should see the correlation between sexual health and proper nutrition. Good wholesome fresh food is vital for building, maintaining, and fueling your sexual system. Following are some additional dietary culprits to avoid.

### Overly Acidic and Overly Alkaline Foods

In our quest to remain sexually vibrant, we need to understand how what we eat affects our internal systems. As already discussed, the human body is predominantly made up of water. The body seeks to maintain its internal environment within certain parameters. When the body becomes too acidic or too alkaline, its internal operations can be severely hampered. When the body produces too much acid, its organ systems lose efficiency. The arteries and veins become less elastic and pliable, and begin to harden. In addition, aging accelerates, the blood pressure increases, the arteries begin to accumulate deposits, and the body starts to lose its ability to rebuild and defend itself.

All of these things can greatly inhibit your effort to remain sexually fit. Sexual problems can also be the result when the body becomes too alkaline. An alkaline internal environment is conducive to many kinds of harmful bacteria, leaving you highly susceptible to yeast and urinary tract infections.

Most of the foods we consume leave a residue when they are broken down into their component parts. Acid foods leave an acid residue, called acid ash, and alkaline foods leave an alkaline residue, called alkaline ash. The best diet to eat to keep acid and alkaline ashes to a minimum focuses on fresh fruits and vegetables. Nutritionally oriented healthcare professionals such as Dr. M. Ted Morter Jr., author of *Your Health, Your Choice* (Lifetime Books, 1993), recommend a diet consisting of 45 percent cooked fruits and vegetables, 30 percent raw fruits and vegetables, and 25 percent grains, nuts, seeds, meat, fish, and poultry.

### High-Fat Meals

Michael T. Murray, N.D., coauthor of *Encyclopedia of Natural Medicine* (Prima Publishing, 1997), says that the quickest way to disrupt your sexual performance is to eat a high-fat meal prior to sexual intercourse. If you have a circulatory problem, you will divert precious blood flow away from your genitals to your digestive system. Your body will have to expend much of its energy and change its blood flow to help digest the fat-laden meal.

## Dead Foods

Are you currently drinking four to five cups of coffee to maintain your energy level and stamina? In between meals, are you loading up on chocolates and other sweets to keep those sugar cravings at bay? Do you consume excessive amounts of salt, soft drinks, fried foods, alcoholic beverages, and fast or processed foods? These foods contain no enzymes, which can be described as the body's workforce. Without an adequate supply of enzymes, metabolic processes and nutrient conversions occur at a slower pace than nature intended. In many cases, the processes shut down due to the faulty enzyme activity.

Excessive salt and sugar also can make the adrenal glands work overtime, as well as cause water retention and high blood pressure. Excessive coffee can cause dehydration. These disorders will definitely affect your sex drive, as your adrenal glands will lose their power to produce the hormones that help to combat stress. And forget trying to maintain an erection under these circumstances. You also will find that your energy levels will dip, as will your sex drive.

A nutritious drink or snack would be better. For example, have a nutritional food bar or drink an 8-ounce glass of water with a teaspoon of whole green food powder (including a variety of green foods such as chlorophyll, barley grass, wheat grass, spirulina, chlorella, and alfalfa). Also, take a 250-milligram capsule of tyrosine.

## Foods for the Sexual Connoisseur

If you consider sex an art form that is renewed with each encounter, please refer to Appendices A, B, and C. There you will find lists of recommended foods, drinks, and books that will help you keep your sex drive in high gear. Also in the chapters that follow you will find an array of information on natural products, detoxification programs, and other natural protocols that assist sexual healing, sexual enjoyment, and emotional satisfaction.

To summarize, you could say that for all intents and purposes, sex begins within, but not without proper nutrition to fuel it or preserve it. Learning how to regulate your food intake to boost your mood and your sex drive can change your life. By taking control of the abundant foods nature offers us, you will not only turn your sex life around, but live a happier and healthier existence.

To ensure that you are properly nourishing your glands, you should:

- Balance your food intake by eating a variety of foods.
- Consume fresh (organic, if possible) fruits and vegetables.
- Consume at least eight 8-ounce glasses of fresh clean water daily.
- Reduce your intake of highly processed foods.
- Consume generous portions of complex carbohydrates, while reducing your intake of sugary snacks and desserts.
- Watch your fat intake. Keep your daily fat consumption to 30 grams or less, with 10 percent coming from unsaturated fatty acids, preferably the omega-3 fatty acids.
- Eat smaller more frequent meals (five to six times a day).
- Reduce or eliminate fried or dead (enzymeless) foods from your diet.
- Reduce your consumption of red meats.
- Reduce your alcohol consumption. Instead, drink more herbal teas and whole green food drinks and juices.
- Take time to relax.
- Reduce your stress load.

And most important, have some sex for dessert tonight!

# 10

# Natural Sex Stimulants

*All too often, even adult conversations about natural aphro-*
*disiacs are accompanied by sly or nervous snickers, and few*
*persons can begin to explain adequately what such sub-*
*stances are or what they do. There exists a vast sea of igno-*
*rance about the subject, a sea that appears to be at flood*
*level.*

Raymond L. McIlvenna, Ph.D.
*The Pleasure Quest: The Search for Aphrodisiacs*
(The Institute for Advanced Study of
Human Sexuality, 1988)

Are there nonmedical substances that can enhance orgasmic pleasure,
increase sensory feelings, increase sex drive, possibly reverse erectile
dysfunction, and improve sexual prowess? How effective are they? Are
they safe? Where can they be obtained? Do they require a prescription?
Can they be taken by individuals on medication? How long do they take
to work?

Answering the questions about natural sex stimulants is the major
goal of this chapter. Since the beginning of time, humans have sought to
discover how foods, plants, water, the sun, and natural elements contribute to health. A large percentage of the medical drugs in use today
are of plant origin. For example, aspirin's active ingredient is derived
from the bark of the white willow tree. Digitalis, the well-known heart
medication, comes from the foxglove plant. Reserpine, a blood pressure
medication, is extracted from an Asian shrub. Ephedrine and pseu-

doephedrine, the active compounds in many cough and cold remedies, are derived from the ephedra plant, a mainstay in Chinese herbology for the last 5,000 years. And vincristine and vinblastine, used to fight the devastating affects of childhood leukemia, comes from the rosy periwinkle tree, prevalent on the Indian Ocean island of Madagascar.

The problem with isolating and mimicking natural compounds lies within the extremely dangerous levels at which medical science uses them. This is why drugs have to go through rigorous testing. The goal, of course, is to find at what level or dose range the drug causes irreparable damage to body tissues and organs.

Present-day thinking centers on the notion that less may be better. In addition, many nonconventional healthcare professionals insist that natural compounds such as the ones just mentioned would better serve the general public if they were used in their natural state.

The trend toward natural remedies is a direct result of the shift toward prevention and away from treatment. While the United States still lags behind other countries, Americans are accepting this change more and more with each passing day. Over the last several years, the trend has also been fueled by several major drugs having been recalled. These recalls were the direct result of deaths associated with the drugs. Among the products recalled were the weight-loss drug fen-phen, the arthritis medication Duract, and the cholesterol fighter cerivastatin. Additionally, Viagra has come under fire for posing serious health complications as well as causing several deaths.

To get a clearer picture of the problem with drugs, please go to http://www.fda.gov/medwatch. Medwatch is the FDA's website for reporting and learning about the safety of medical products. It includes reports on recalls of and safety issues concerning medical drugs. David Allison, Ph.D., a professor in the Department of Biostatistics and the Clinical Nutrition Research Center at the University of Alabama at Bimingham, reminds us that all drugs and pharmacologically active substances can cause side effects. He insists that we should not only be aware of them, but take them seriously.

The combination of wanting to avoid possibly dangerous drugs and being drawn to natural compounds that gently modulate the body's functions rather than overriding them is what is driving this current trend toward alternative remedies. As part of this movement, people are turning to natural sexual performance enhancers as their first choice over medical remedies. In the following pages, we will review the accessory nutrients, amino acids, enzymes, herbs, hormones, vitamins, minerals, green foods, and phytochemicals that are currently in popular use.

## Accessory Nutrients

Accessory nutrients are compounds that are important to health but that cannot be classified as a vitamin, mineral, or herb. While many accessory nutrients are not required by the body, they have specific actions that can help you improve your general health as well as restore, maintain, or improve your sexual health and performance. Four accessory nutrients that are commonly used to combat sexual problems are colostrum, deer antler, evening primrose oil, and letchin.

### Colostrum

When we are born, we enter the world with an untested immune system. Our tiny bodies must immediately defend us against the countless assaults that each day brings. It is from our mother's first breast milk that we receive a natural substance that provides us with the factors responsible for building our immunity and natural resistance. That substance is colostrum. Colostrum is actually a nonmilk compound that is secreted by the mammary gland in the later stages of pregnancy. These secretions intensify right before birth and cease within two to three days following it. Lance S. Wright, M.D., founder of the American Holistic Medical Association and a professor of integrative medicine at the Capital University of Integrative Medicine in Washington, D.C., says that "this first meal of babies is the perfect combination of all the necessary immune and growth factors." He adds that the ingredients in colostrum work to activate more than fifty different physical processes in the newborn body, hence colostrum's designation as life's first food.

Currently the evidence is mounting that the array of components found in colostrum such as immunoglobulins, lymphokines, lactoferrin, cytokines, and interleukins offer the same benefits to adults in supplemental form. It is this feature as well as the high content of immunoglobulin 7 ($IgG_7$), insulin-like growth factors, and growth hormones that make colostrum a viable aid in safeguarding your sexual health. Also by supplying necessary nutrients like human growth hormone that fuel or stimulate the sexual communication system, colostrum can greatly contribute to your efforts to remain healthy and sexually vibrant.

*Additional Benefits*
None.

*Suggested Dose*
Follow the manufacturer's guidelines.

## Deer Antler

The last several decades have seen a growing interest in the medicinal value of deer antlers. Yes, deer antlers—those funny-looking things on the top of Rudolph the Red Nose Reindeer's head! Studies conducted on the biochemistry of deer antlers have found that they contain a very interesting natural compound that can improve sexual performance, stamina, and strength. All of the excitement surrounding this substance, known as velvet, centers on the ability of deer antler to regenerate itself. Deer antler is one of only a very small pool of mammalian organs that have this capability. Used for more than 2,000 years in China, deer antler is revered for its ability to promote wellness and has served as a restorative aid in a number of illnesses. Its hallmark feature is its ability to protect and regulate normal bodily processes, although it has few curative powers.

New research out of the University of Alberta in Canada has substantiated many of the long-term traditional uses of deer antler, such as:

- Reducing cholesterol levels.
- Stimulating a strong immune response.
- Lowering the blood pressure.
- Reducing inflammation and the negative effects of arthritis.
- Improving athletic performance.

Part of what keeps the sexual communication system primed is the body's production of growth hormone and insulin-like growth factors (IGFs). These substances are intimately connected to testosterone (the hormone of desire), and deer antler has high amounts of each. Both insulin-like growth factors 1 and 2, which play major roles in the proper growth and function of most organs in the body, contain insulin. Because aging causes a decline in these chemicals, which modulate the sexual appetite, supplementation with velvet has been shown to rekindle lost sex drive, stamina, and the raw sexual appetite usually attributed to youth. Scientists in Asia, China, and Russia, where much of the research has been conducted, suggest that deer antler, or velvet, stimulates production of the hormones that are vital to sexual health and functioning. Furthermore, owing to its ability to improve circulation and reduce cholesterol deposits, deer antler is used extensively to treat impotency and disorders resulting in decreased blood flow to the pelvic cavity in both males and females.

### Additional Benefits

- Improves lung function.
- Improves circulation.
- Tones muscle and glandular tissues.
- Increases the ratio of collagen, chondrocytes, and glycosaminoglycans (chondroitin sulfate), which are essential to good joint health.
- Reduces stress.
- Restores the energy levels to normal.

### Suggested Dose

Follow the manufacturer's guidelines.

## Evening Primrose Oil

The evening primrose has a storied history and in recent years has been the subject of intense investigation. The plant got its name because its bright yellow flowers look like primrose flowers and because it blooms in the evening. What makes the plant so unique is that it is not really a primrose or part of the primrose species. Rather, it belongs to the willow herb family and is more of a weed than a plant. The remarkable thing about the evening primrose is that it grows wild along roadsides and on waste sites, and thrives even in places like sand dunes, according to Judy Graham, author of *Evening Primrose Oil* (Thorsons Publishers, 1984). Many of its health-giving benefits come from its oil being converted in the body to a substance known as prostaglandin $E_1$. ($PGE_1$). $PGE_1$ is used to alleviate the symptoms associated with health conditions such as PMS, cirrhosis of the liver, benign breast disease, heart disease, and vascular dysfunction.

Prostaglandins were first discovered in 1935 by Ulf S. von Euler, a Swedish scientist. Von Euler named his newly found molecules "prostaglandins" because they are found in abundance in the seminal fluid. He believed it originates in the prosthetic fluid of the prostate gland.

Like the hormonal system, prostaglandins control and modulate many of the body's functions. However, they do not act like the hormones, traveling to remote sites, turning biological functions on and off. Rather, they stay put and control the operations of each and every cell in their area. However, they are everywhere, in blood vessel walls, platelets, nerve fibers, immune system, and every organ in the body. Sexually, $PGE_1$ controls the effects of estrogen, progesterone, and prolactin as well as influencing adrenal function and behavior, the latter via its regulation of the brain neurotransmitters.

Oil of evening primrose is also rich in substances called gamma-linolenic acid and linoleic acid, two important essential fatty acids.

### Additional Benefits

- Helps treat multiple sclerosis (MS).
- Has anti-inflammatory effects.
- Protects and insulates the nerve fibers.
- Cushions and protects the body tissues.
- Alleviates chronic fatigue.

### Suggested Dose
Follow the manufacturer's guidelines.

## Letchin

Letchin is abundant in the human body. Historically, letchin is used to assist the body in its efforts to emulsify dietary fat. It is also used in many European countries to boost sexual vitality, as it is involved in proper sex hormone secretion. An added benefit of letchin supplementation is its positive effect on brain and nerve function, due to its role in the health of the neurotransmitters. Letchin also has high concentrations of phosphatidylcholine, which affects the vitality of brain hormone secretions, the sex drive, and sexual arousal.

*Additional Benefits*

- Lowers the cholesterol levels.
- Prevents hardening of the arteries.
- Prevents the accumulation of fatty deposits in the liver.
- Increases memory retention.
- Improves brain function.
- Improves digestion.
- Energizes the sexual glands.

*Suggested Dose*
Follow the manufacturer's guidelines.

## Amino Acids

To many in the bodybuilding world, amino acids are very well known and are used extensively. They are the basic building blocks of protein. There are twenty-two known amino acids, with eight classified as "essential" and fourteen as nonessential. (See Table 10.1.) The essential

### TABLE 10.1.
### THE TWENTY-TWO AMINO ACIDS

| Essential | |
| --- | --- |
| Isoleucine | Phenylalanine |
| Leucine | Threonine |
| Lysine | Tryptophan |
| Methionine | Valine |

| Nonessential Amino Acids | |
| --- | --- |
| Alanine | Glutathione |
| Arginine | Glycine |
| Aspartic acid | Histidine |
| Carnitine | Proline |
| Cysteine | Serine |
| Glutamic acid | Taurine |
| Glutamine | Tyrosine |

amino acids must be obtained from the diet because they are not manufactured by the body. The nonessential amino acids are manufactured by the body and therefore not necessary in the diet. Amino acids are formed as a direct result of food being metabolized. Specifically, they are the end result of protein metabolism.

The amino acids exert a powerful influence on a number of biological systems. The designations "essential" and "nonessential" are actually misleading. We need all 22 of the amino acids. The body uses all of them to construct the molecules that compose it. Without the aminos the body could not rebuild or repair itself.

Researchers now know that not only are the amino acids vital in overall health maintenance, but specific ones have shown specific abilities. Dr. Arnold Pike, former director of the Academy of Nutritional Sciences, says, "While they are the building blocks of which proteins are constructed and are the end-products of digestion, specific functions have been found for some of these amino acids that play a vital role in your health." Among the amino acids that have the ability to enhance sexual capabilities are the following:

## Carnosine

Carnosine is a naturally occurring combination of the amino acid alanine and histamine, a compound released during allergic reactions. It has very powerful antioxidant and immune-boosting capabilities. It also appears to promote wound healing as well as reduce inflammation due to its ability to help regulate adrenal gland function. In addition, carnosine has powerful antiaging capabilities and slows down one of the processes that accelerates aging the most—glycosylation. Glycosylation causes cross-linking, which has been attributed with damaging dioxyribonucleic acid (DNA) molecules (your genetic blueprint) and forming deviant proteins.

In 1956 Denham Harman, M.D., Ph.D., formulated the free radical theory of aging. Simply put, Dr. Harman found that certain molecules have the ability to randomly cause cell damage and accelerate aging. These molecules attack the cellular membranes, alter the DNA, cause lipid peroxidation (the formation of rancid fats), and decrease the immune response. In other words, the body mistakes its own tissues as foreign invaders and makes an all-out assault. Invariably, the individual suffers pain, inflammation, and a host of other negative symptoms.

The cross-linking of proteins only adds to the fiasco as the molecules become so tightly entangled that they start to intersect. As the process continues, pain, stiffness, and decreased mobility of the joints can occur. Eventually the connective tissue, called collagen, begins to lose its elasticity and flexibility, which affects not only overall health, but also sexuality. As the internal aging process accelerates, so does the decline of the sexual communication system. Carnosine plays a major role in slowing down these processes of glycosylation and cross-linking.

### Additional Benefits

- Boosts the libido and the sex drive.
- Prevents muscle fatigue.
- Helps to slow down corneal erosion.
- Protects the neural tissues.
- Protects against the kidney and neuropathy complications associated with diabetes.

### Suggested Dose
Take 50 to 100 milligrams daily.

### Note
Carnosine and carnitine are not the same thing. Please do not confuse the two.

---

### SPECIAL NOTE

Most of the amino acids come in two forms: a D-form and an L-form. The two forms are mirror images of each other, with the chemical structure of the L-form spiraling to the left (the "L" stands for *levo,* which is Latin for "left") and the chemical structure of the D-form spiraling to the right (the "D" stands for *dextro,* which is Latin for "right"). In general, the L-form is better absorbed and assimilated in human tissue than the D-form. Therefore, use supplements containing the L-forms of the amino acids (except for methionine and phenylalanine), and avoid supplements that contain only the D-forms. Methionine and phenylalanine can also be found in a third form, the DL-form, which is a mixture of the D- and L-forms. In these two amino acids, and only these two, the D-forms are converted to the L-forms within the body, making the DL-forms metabolically effective.

## L-Arginine

Arginine is highly touted for its ability to stimulate growth hormone release in the pituitary gland. Because it also functions in protein synthesis, it has become popular in bodybuilding circles. In addition, according to research conducted by Jacob Rajfer, M.D., a urologist at the University of California at Los Angeles, and colleagues, arginine is the precursor of nitric oxide, which helps to widen the blood vessels and regulate blood flow. Based on their research, Dr. Rajfer and his colleagues said in their report in the *New England Journal of Medicine* in 1992 that 80 percent of the problems associated with impotency in the United States are a direct result of faulty nitric oxide production. So important is nitric oxide to the function of the smooth muscles within the arteries that it was declared the molecule of the year in 1992 by the editors of *Science* magazine.

Arthur L. Burnett, M.D., of Johns Hopkins Hospital in Baltimore, in his research also found that arginine is what regulates nitric oxide production. Dr. Burnett maintains that nitric oxide mediates many of the different mechanisms involved in sustaining a proper erection. Furthermore, according to Timothy Maher, Ph.D., professor of pharmaceutical sciences and dean of research and sponsored programs at the Massachusetts College of Pharmacy and Health Sciences, "The best correlated biochemical marker for predicting vascular dysfunction appears to be the ratio of L-Arginine to 'ADMA' in plasma."

ADMA, or asymmetric dimethy-L-arginine, is a substance that slows down nitric oxide production.

### Additional Benefits

- Increases immune function.
- Promotes good cardiovascular health.
- Helps heal burns.
- Stabilizes the blood pressure.
- Increases the circulation.
- Stimulates growth hormone production.

### Suggested Dose

Take 1 to 4 grams daily.

## L-Carnitine

Carnitine is used as a fat burner and an aid in increasing the energy levels. Researchers have found it to be very beneficial in alleviating the symptoms of chronic fatigue syndrome. One of carnitine's major functions is in the disposal of triglycerides via the mitochondria. The mitochondria are tiny energy factories within the cells where the body converts carbohydrates, fats, and proteins into fuel. Carnitine transports fats into the mitochondria, which helps to improve the energy levels, control weight, maintain good heart health, and sustain proper cholesterol levels.

Carnitine also affects sexual performance through its effects on sperm. As you know, sperm cells are produced in the testes, but are not fully developed there. It is within the epididymis that the sperm mature and develop the capability to fertilize the female egg. Researchers have found that men who are infertile have extremely low levels of carnitine in their semen. Supplemental carnitine has been shown to increase the motility of the sperm cells, improving their chance of reaching the female egg.

### Additional Benefits

- Increases athletic performance.
- Prevents cirrhosis of the liver.
- Reduces triglyceride levels.
- Increases HDL levels.
- Improves muscle strength.
- Stimulates the metabolism of the branched-chain amino acids in the skeletal system for energy during extended periods of exercise.

### Suggested Dose
Take 500 milligrams daily.

### SPECIAL NOTE

Many of the amino acids are responsible for constructing, repairing, and modulating the neurotransmitters. Since neurotransmitter activity is intimately linked to the sexual communication system, it would be wise to add a full-range amino acid supplement to your sexual health regimen.

## Glutamine

Glutamine is probably best known for its ability to heal the body and increase protein synthesis. It is used to speed up the healing of wounds and to aid in the recovery of burn victims. In addition, while glucose serves as the brain's preferred fuel source, glutamine is the fuel that runs the immune system.

According to J. D. Fernstrom, Ph.D., a professor of psychiatry, pharmacology, and behavioral neuroscience at the University of Pittsburgh's School of Medicine, glutamine is found in high concentrations in the central nervous system. Here it functions as an excitatory neurotransmitter, a substance vital to maintaining mental and sexual vitality. Furthermore, glutamine is also used as a fuel source in the brain, where it increases mental alertness and acts to combat depression. This is due in part to its serving as a substrate for gamma amino butyric acid (GABA), a natural tranquilizer.

Supplemental glutamine helps the body maintain its proper pH levels. It is currently used in hospital settings to protect the liver from the negative effects of chemotherapy.

### Additional Benefits

- Serves as the primary source of fuel for the cells of the intestinal tract.
- Promotes lean tissue growth.
- Protects the brain from ammonia toxicity.
- Functions as a powerful antioxidant.
- Controls the blood sugar levels.

### Suggested Dose

Take 1,000 to 4,000 milligrams in two equal dosages daily.

## Tyrosine

Known as the feel-good amino acid, tyrosine can leave you highly energized and in a mood ready for love. Tyrosine acts as a mood elevator. Researchers in the Department of Neuroscience at the University of Milan School of Medicine in Italy found that tyrosine plays a major role in the synthesis of dopamine and norepinephrine, two brain chemicals involved with modulating the sex drive, sexual appetite, and overall alertness. It is also involved in the production of adrenaline and noradrenaline by the adrenal glands. Tyrosine will give you back your sexual mood as it alleviates your stress, calms your nerves, and lifts your spirits.

### Additional Benefits

- Combats chronic fatigue syndrome.
- Assists in proper thyroid function.
- Prevents mental fatigue.

### Suggested Dose
Take 300 to 600 milligrams twice daily.

### Note
Tyrosine can also be purchased as acetyl-tyrosine, a stabler form that is recommended due to its ability to better penetrate the blood-brain barrier.

# Herbs

Dr. Edward E. Shook in his epic masterpiece *Advanced Treatise in Herbology* (Trinity Center Press, 1978) defines herbalism, also called herbology, as the branch of science that deals with the therapeutic properties of herbs. Dr. Shook states that "every disease known to human kind is primarily a condition of unbalanced chemical constituents of both elements and compounds which compose the tissues and fluids of the whole system." In his estimation, bombarding the body with drugs or other agents that cannot be utilized by the cells will further disrupt or interfere with the body's attempt to heal itself. This is the reason for the many side effects and safety issues associated with long-term drug use. While helping to control or alleviate one problem, another is caused. For example, while treating diabetes, liver and kidney damage occur. Dr Shook says that although the reason is not understood, "herbs can and do assimilate inorganic mineral matter." He adds:

> Though some mysterious and unknown alchemy herbs convert this inert and lifeless matter into living organic material which when presented to the animal or human cell, is hungrily absorbed, sustaining and renewing life's process.

In this section we will look at the herbs that are commonly used today to treat sexual dysfunction.

## Damiana

Damiana is found in the Mexican Gulf and parts of South America. Revered for its ability to stimulate the central nervous system, damiana is used as a tonic that promotes well-being. Touted as a rejuvenator of both the male and the female sexual systems, it has been found to contain many alkaloids that affect sex organ function and sensory feeling. This makes it extremely valuable in treating females suffering from frigidity. Damiana is also hailed for its ability to restore lost libido by stimulating testosterone production. In addition, it produces a mild euphoric feeling, which promotes contentment and thus removes inhibitions. When using damiana in tea form, add a teaspoon of catnip tea to the cup of damiana tea. Anecdotally this intensifies the euphoric effect of damiana.

### Additional Benefits

- Increases the sperm count.
- Restores sexual capabilities when combinned with saw palmetto.
- Relieves constipation.
- Acts as an antidepressant.
- Relieves headaches.
- Treats dysmenorrhea (painful menstruation).
- Treats nephritis (kidney inflammation).

### Suggested Dose

Follow the manufacturer's guidelines. Earl Mindell, Ph.D., recommends no more than three tablets daily. Take damiana on an off-and-on cycle— for example three weeks on and one month off.

### Note

In Mexico, damiana is used by doctors to treat inflammation of the bladder, orchitis (inflammation of the testicles), and spermatorrhea (involuntary explosions of sperm).

## Don Quai

Don quai is one of the herbs most widely used by females. Employed extensively in Asia for more than 2,000 years, it contains phytoestrogens, which are effective at alleviating hot flashes, night sweats, and other symptoms related to menopause. Also known as angelica, don quai grows in China, Korea, and Japan. In traditional Chinese medicine it has long been considered the queen of herbs. *Don quai* is Chinese for "you are compelled to return." This refers to the herb's ability to normalize female bodily functions that have gone awry. Also widely used in the United States, don quai is considered an all-purpose toning herb for women with the ability to:

- Increase the blood flow to the genitals.
- Balance the hormonal cycles.
- Alleviate menstrual irregularities.
- Strengthen liver and kidney function.
- Stimulate uterine contractions during childbirth.
- Restore vaginal lubrication.
- Strengthen the reproductive organs.
- Alleviate migraine headaches that occur during menopause.
- Eliminate the atrophy of the vaginal tissue that often occurs during menopause.

Herbal researchers have isolated several agents in don quai that have antispasmodic and vasodilation properties. These are the features that researchers claim make don quai an excellent synergistic herb, assisting other substances via its circulatory actions.

### Additional Benefits

- Normalizes the blood pressure.
- Purifies the blood.
- Reduces blood clotting.
- Increases production of the sex hormones in both males and females.
- Relieves constipation.
- Has antiviral and antitumor properties.

*Suggested Dose*
Follow the manufacturer's guidelines.

*Note*
Don quai should not be used during pregnancy or menstruation.

While don quai is considered mainly a female herb, it is used by males as a blood purifier and to jump-start waning hormone production.

## Ginko Biloba

Ginko biloba is primarily used today for its ability to increase the circulation, especially to the brain. Because of this ability, it is touted as a memory booster. Ginko has also been found by researchers in Europe and China to be highly effective at improving the circulation to the genitals. Its effectiveness at boosting the circulation is attributed to substances called flavone glycosides and ginkolides, which prevent the platelets from clumping together. In some individuals, ginko has increased the intensity and duration of orgasms.

*Additional Benefits*

- Increases the circulation to all the parts of the body via the capillaries.
- Promotes oxygen production.
- Treats tinnitus (ringing in the ears).
- Helps against Alzheimer's disease.
- Combats lung and asthma disorders.
- Counteracts the effects of diarrhea.

*Suggested Dose*
Take 40 to 50 milligrams of a standardized extract containing 24 percent flavone glycosides and 6 percent ginkolides, three times daily.

## Ginseng

Ginseng is probably the most well-known herb in the United States. Made popular by Russian athletes in the Olympics, ginseng is revered for its ability to increase energy and stamina, as well as improve mental concentration. Classified as an adaptogen, ginseng has remarkable powers in helping the body adapt to stress. As a sexual stimulant, it has been used extensively in China since the sixteenth century. Still used today to enhance sexual performance, it stimulates the formation of healthy cells in both the male and the female reproductive organs. For this reason, ginseng is often referred to as the "root of life."

Additionally, ginseng has shown the ability to increase nitric oxide synthesis, thus benefitting the health and flexibility of the penile blood vessels and modulating blood flow. To enhance sexual performance, take ginseng one to two hours before intercourse.

### Additional Benefits

- Promotes sex hormone production in both males and females.
- Acts as a powerful immune and antiviral stimulant.
- Decreases the blood pressure.
- Reduces the cholesterol levels.
- Alleviates the symptoms of menopause.
- Stabilizes the blood sugar levels.

### Suggested Dose

Take 300 to 400 milligrams a day of Siberian ginseng or 100 to 200 milligrams a day of panax ginseng.

### Note

Ginseng comes in different varieties. The most common are American ginseng (*Panax quinquefolium*), Chinese or Korean ginseng (*Panax ginseng*), and Siberian ginseng (*Eleutherococcus senticosus*). All of these varieties promote energy and stamina, but Korean ginseng is the most stimulating for immediate needs.

## Horny Goat Weed

What a fantastic name! Horny goat weed was first discovered by Chinese farmers who noticed that aging goats were sexually revived after consuming what were described as large, thorn-covered weeds that other animals would not eat. Although researchers are still unsure of exactly how horny goat weed works, the Chinese farmers' observation gave birth to the herb's now famous and hilarious name. Researchers have determined, however, horny goat weed's action centers on testosterone production. They believe that the herb inactivates an enzyme called acetylcholinesterase (ACHE). ACHE inactivates the cholinergic neuro-transmitters in the brain that increase sexual arousal.

In both sexes, horny goat weed increases the sexual appetite, stimulates the sensory nerves, and acts like testosterone, boosting the sex drive, the libido, and stamina. In females horny goat weed alleviates menstrual discomfort. Also known as epimedium and yin yang hou, the herb is regularly used by doctors in Shanghai. Dr. Diao Yuan Kuang of Shanghai's Longhua Hospital says that the herb returns sexual strength. This powerful herb is also recommended for use by the Chinese Academy of Sciences. The various forms of horny goat weed sold in the United States are blends of natural ingredients that work synergistically to improve sexual performance and increase the natural sexual capacity.

### Additional benefits

- Increases energy and stamina.
- Combats aging.
- Stimulates the nerves throughout the genital area.
- Supports normal prostate, kidney, and liver function.

### Suggested Dose
Follow the manufacturer's guidelines.

### Note
In a double-blind, placebo-controlled study by Steven Lamm, M.D., sexual satisfaction was found to be greatly enhanced in 60 percent of the healthy males participating in the study. The results were similar to those of 45 percent of the men taking Viagra. In the study, the men taking horny goat weed were given 1,616 milligrams daily for three months. Two hours prior to sexual intercourse, they took an additional 3,232 milligrams.

## Maca

Maca is causing quite a stir in the natural health industry. From Peru, it is known as Peruvian ginseng, although it is not a member of the ginseng family. It is used in South America by physicians to treat male impotency, hot flashes, infertility, vaginal dryness, and a host of other problems.

Researchers have found that maca stimulates the pituitary gland, known as the master gland. Two natural active components in maca, P-methoxybenzyl isothiocyanate and aromatic isothiocyanates, have strong aphrodisiac properties. The benefits of the herb, found in animal studies and published in the April 2000 issue of the journal *Urology*, include promoting an increase in libido, sexual potency, and energy.

Extensively used for decades by Peruvian medical doctors, the herb has also been personally used by Gary F. Gordon, M.D., the former president of the American College for Advancement in Medicine. From his personal experience, Dr. Gordon cites improved erectile tissue response. He insists that maca can be used to help regulate the production of the steroid hormones such as testosterone, progesterone, and estrogen. Dr. Gordon, who now practices in Chicago, adds that "maca restores men to a more healthy functional status in which they experience a more active libido."

### Additional Benefits

- Inhibits osteoporosis.
- Promotes immune system functioning.
- Enhances overall energy and stamina.
- Influences proper adrenal, thyroid, and pancreatic function.
- Balances hormone production.

### Suggested Dose
Take 4 grams daily.

## Muira Puama

Used for centuries by the natives of Brazil to rejuvenate the libido and sexual desire, muira puama is just beginning to work its way into mainstream America. Muria puama is a highly touted sexual stimulant. Natural sterols found within the herb, including beta-sitosterol, a compound popular among bodybuilders, are believed to give muira puama its aphrodisiac properties. The results of studies conducted in France included the restoration of libido and the reversal of impotency in more than 62 percent of the individuals who used the herb. The French researchers also found that 51 percent of the males who used the herb successfully attained erections. Muira puama is also known as potency wood.

### Additional Benefits

- Increases the strength of the genital muscles.
- Prolongs erections.
- Treats disorders of the nervous system.
- Alleviates menstrual cramps.
- Improves circulation.
- Combats rheumatism.
- Relieves gastrointestinal distress.
- Promotes endurance.
- Heightens sensory awareness.

### Suggested Dose

Take 2 to 4 grams daily. Use only as needed.

## Yohimbe

Yohimbe is one of the most common herbs used to treat impotency. Cultivated in Africa, yohimbe is used extensively in the United States. Its active ingredient, called yohimbine, is used by many urologists to treat erectile dysfunction. Yohimbe works by dilating the blood vessels, thus allowing increased blood flow to the erectile chambers in the penis. Before the introduction of Viagra, this herb, as yohimbine hydrochloride, was the only FDA-approved medication to treat erectile dysfunction. The dosage is usually about 5.4 milligrams three times daily. A much weaker form of yohimbe is available over-the-counter, but in very low dosages. When using over-the-counter yohimbe, divide your intake into equal dosages taken throughout the day.

Yohimbe also stimulates the central nervous system, which helps to increase the sex drive and libido. Because of this, yohimbe is also used to treat sexual arousal disorder in women. Dr. David Mobley has found 16.2 milligrams of yohimbe taken in divided dosages before sexual intercourse to be highly effective.

*Additional Benefits*

- Blocks alpha-adrenoreceptors, thus diminishing the effect of hormones that constrict the blood vessels as a result of aging.
- Discourages vascular leakage.
- Prolongs sexual stamina by delaying ejaculation.
- Treats premature ejaculation.
- Boosts pleasurable sensations.
- Improves stamina and energy levels.

*Suggested Dose*
Follow the manufacturer's guidelines. Do not exceed the recommended dose levels.

*Note*
Yohimbe is a monoamine oxidase (MAO) inhibitor and should not be used by individuals taking antidepressant medication or by individuals suffering from poorly controlled blood pressure. In addition, do not take yohimbe if you have liver or heart disease.

## Other Herbal Sex Stimulants

In addition to the eight herbs just discussed, the following herbs also function as sexual stimulants.

- *Cayenne.* Cayenne is known for its highly stimulative properties, which are attributed to its capsaicin content. It improves circulation throughout the body, efficiently moving blood to depressed genitals.
- *Garlic.* Garlic is excellent for controlling high blood pressure. It reduces or eliminates plaque buildup around arterial tissue and has strong immune and antiviral properties. It keeps the sex glands toned and energized and can increase the sperm count.
- *Gotu Kola.* Gotu kola is an excellent tonic. It is useful in cases of improper blood flow and stamina.
- *Licorice.* Licorice is a very popular herb that is used for its tonic effects. It is beneficial for relieving adrenal gland exhaustion. Similar in composition to the hormones found in the adrenal cortex, it has anti-inflammatory and immune-stimulating properties.

It also can normalize menstrual irregularities related to decreased progesterone levels, as well as detox the liver. However, licorice should be taken with care. It can raise the blood pressure due to its stimulating effects. Look for the uralenis variety rather than the *Glycyrrhiza glabra* type. The alkaloid glabra is what raises the blood pressure. Also look for labels that say "deglycyrrhized."

- *Pygeum.* Pygeum is used extensively with saw palmetto to alleviate the symptoms of an enlarged prostate gland. It is also used to help restore potency in males incapable of sustaining erections.

- *Sarsaparilla.* This well-known herb has been used as a blood purifier. As a central nervous system stimulant, it combats anxiety and tension. It stimulates the production of the sex hormones, and revitalizes diminished sexual desire.

- *Tribulus Terrestis.* Tribulus terrestis is very popular with the bodybuilding community for its ability to increase stamina, strength, and the androgen testosterone. It is used extensively in India to treat impotency and to stimulate the libido in both men and women. Dr. Howard Peiper and Nina Anderson state in *Natural Solutions for Sexual Dysfunction* (Safe Goods, 1998) that tribulus benefits the endocrine system and hormone production due to its actions in the liver, where it breaks down fat and cholesterol to make hormones.

- *Wild Oats.* Wild oats is also known in natural health circles as *Avena sativa.* It is used primarily to boost the sex drive, libido, and sexual desire. It is also used to stimulate natural testosterone production. *Avena sativa* is used by both genders.

In addition, there are a number of herbs that help disorders such as diabetes, low energy, low stamina, stress, hormonal imbalance, immunity, and cholesterol levels, which affect sexuality. They include:

| | |
|---|---|
| • Ashwangandha | • Fo-ti |
| • Astragalus | • Ginger |
| • Black cohosh | • Guarana |
| • Blessed thistle | • Gymnema sylvestre |
| • Bilberry | • Kava kava |
| • Bitter mellow | • Nettle |
| • Chinese morinda root | • Wild yams |
| • Fenugreek | • Withania |

When deciding on which individual or combination of natural sex stimulants to try, choose a product that addresses your unique needs and biochemistry. Ask yourself, "What is my specific problem—potency, arousal, diminished sex drive, stress, hormones, or premature ejaculation?"

Then choose a product that will help solve that problem. The biggest mistake individuals make is basing their choice on what worked for their sister, brother, best girlfriend, or buddy. Do a little homework and make sure the ingredients will address your specific needs. When choosing a natural sex stimulant, remember that "one size does not fit all."

## Hormones

Hormones are the chemical messengers that fuel your sexual nature and sensuality. Once you understand how to utilize hormones, you could well be on your way to solving many of your problems related to sexual decline. Dr. Hans Selye feels that a breakdown in the processes connected to the hormones can spell disaster. Restoring youthful sexuality may just be a matter of restoring your levels of these powerful substances to what they were during your younger years. This point is echoed by Dr. William Regelson, coauthor of *The Superhormone Promise* (Simon & Schuster, 1996):

> At a certain point, usually around age forty-five to fifty, melatonin levels start to significantly decline. This in turn sends a signal to the rest of the superhormones and to the other body systems that you have crossed the threshold, and the aging process begins. The good news is that we believe it is possible to reset the aging clock and to slow down and even reverse the aging process by restoring our superhormone levels to their youthful peaks.

In this section, we will discuss the hormones connected with our sexual health and how to use them to restore our youthful sensuality.

### Androstendione

Androstendione is a precursor to testosterone, the male hormone responsible for increasing the sex drive and libido. It is very popular with the bodybuilding community and was made famous by Mark McGwire of the St. Louis Cardinals. However, because of how quickly the body breaks down the hormone and because the hormone is also a direct precursor to estrogen, it may not be the best testosterone booster to kickstart a sluggish libido, according to Dr. Carlton M. Colker.

### Additional Benefits
None.

### Suggested Dose
Follow the manufacturer's guidelines. To heighten sexual arousal, stamina, and possibly performance, use shortly before sexual activity.

## DHEA

Dehydroepiandrosterone (DHEA) is the most abundant steroid hormone within the human body. It is intimately involved with adrenal function and therefore responsible for controlling the body's ability to adapt to stress, as well as its manufacture of the sex hormones. Studies have demonstrated conclusively that levels of this hormone decline sharply as aging progresses. By age 60, the body makes only about 10 to 20 percent of what it did at age 25. In experiments, supplemental DHEA has shown the ability the extend the life span of laboratory animals.

Produced by the adrenal glands, DHEA is not found in any food. Most of the DHEA that is commercially sold is made synthetically using Mexican wild yams. Researchers believe that DHEA plays a role in the mechanisms involved with proper erections, and increases sexual appetite and performance. Dubbed the fountain of youth hormone, DHEA has shown the ability to slow down age-related changes in sexuality, cognitive recall, energy levels, and general overall health.

### Additional Benefits

- Modulates testosterone and estrogen production.
- Enhances immune function.
- Assists the body in maintaining lean muscle.
- Increases $IGF_1$ production.
- Stimulates the production of cholecystokin (CCK), which controls the appetite.
- Modulates glucose metabolism.

***Suggested Dose***
Take 5 to 10 milligrams daily.

***Note***
Do not take DHEA if you have a hormone-related cancer such as breast, ovarian, or prostate cancer.

Have your DHEA levels tested before adding the hormone to your supplement program.

## Estrogen

As we learned in Chapter 2, estrogen is the predominant hormone found in women. It is the hormone that makes a woman a woman. Women's bodies actually produce three forms of estrogen—estradiol, estrone, and estriol. Estradiol is believed to be the most stimulating form, causing the most problems, such as breast cancer. Estriol is the weakest form but is believed to be the most protective.

When we think of estrogen therapy, we usually think of its use to relieve the symptoms associated with menopause such as:

- Vaginal dryness
- Loss of libido
- Night sweats
- Hot flashes
- Loss of short-term memory
- Increased irritability
- Moodiness
- Frequent vaginal infections

Some other problems associated with declining estrogen levels are:

- Weight gain
- Joint pain
- Increased risk of heart disease and heart attack
- Elevated serum cholesterol levels
- Loss of bone density, osteoporosis
- Increased risk of developing Alzheimer's disease

To combat many of these negative changes, medical doctors have for years prescribed estrogen, primarily in the form of Premarin, which is extracted from the urine of horses. This treatment has been very effective, also returning the women to their youthful, premenopausal state. Estrogen can be administered either orally or through skin patches that are usually changed twice a week. However, there are risks involved. Estrogen replacement therapy (ERT) has been linked to:

- High blood pressure
- Breast cancer (if taken for 10 to 20 years)
- Endometrial cancer (when taken alone—that is, without progesterone, the other dominant female hormone)
- Fibroid tumors

For some women, the long-term complications and side effects can make ERT a very unviable choice. Therefore, many healthcare professionals today advocate the use of weaker, milder phytoestrogens. Phytoestrogens are found naturally in various plants and herbs. They have been used extensively by Asian women for centuries. Research has clearly shown that these women suffer from fewer complications associated with PMS and menopause. Among the plants and herbs that contain phytoestrogens are the following:

- Astragalus
- Black cohosh
- Blue cohosh
- Chasteberry
- Damiana
- Don quai
- Evening primrose oil
- Licorice root
- Motherwort
- Red clover
- Sage
- Soy
- Vervain
- Wild yams

In addition, there are numerous natural estrogen and progesterone creams and sprays that can be purchased without a doctor's prescription.

### Additional Benefits

- Has growth hormone capabilities.
- Raises the HDL cholesterol levels.
- Protects against fibroid tumors.
- Stabilizes the blood sugar levels.

- Decreases the anticlotting factors.
- Controls problems related to incontinence.

### Suggested Dose

Follow your doctor's orders or the manufacturer's guidelines, depending on the particular product you use.

### Note

ERT must be monitored by a qualified healthcare professional. If you prefer to use a natural hormone replacement product, you should still first discuss it with your healthcare provider.

If you have a family history of breast or endometrial cancer, you should avoid estrogen replacement therapy.

## Human Growth Hormone

Over the last several decades there has been an explosion of information concerning human growth hormone (HGH). Secreted by the pituitary gland, HGH is a youth hormone. HGH supplementation has been shown to help restore vigor, sexual stamina, and libido. Additionally, it has shown the ability to help restore vaginal lubrication, in essence returning the vaginal tissue to its soft, pliable, elastic state.

After being released, HGH is transported to the liver and converted into a protein called somatomedin C, also known as insulin-like growth factor 1 ($IGF_1$). It is $IGF_1$ that is partially responsible for the growth hormone function in the body. In fact, Ronald Katz, M.D., president of the American Academy of Anti-Aging Medicine, reminds us that $IGF_1$ is actually more important that HGH itself. Dr. Katz says that the levels of HGH can vary widely throughout the day. The levels decline steadily after age 30, and researchers estimate that more than half of the population is deficient by age 65. Decreased HGH is linked to:

- Increased aging.
- Decreased immunity.
- Increased cholesterol levels.
- Reduced energy and stamina.
- Decrease in lean muscle tissue.
- Loss of libido.

The first study on the positive effects of HGH supplementation was published in 1990 in the *New England Journal of Medicine*. Researchers at the Medical College of Wisconsin in Milwaukee found a marked reduction in adipose tissue and an increase in bone density. In the study participants who took HGH replacement therapy has also been shown to increase the intensity of orgasms, especially in aging females. Males have found an improvement in sex drive, vigor, and sexual performance. Increased mental clarity and memory have been found in both sexes.

### Additional Benefits

- Reduces menopausal symptoms.
- Improves mental focus.
- Improves glucose metabolism.
- Adjusts the muscle-to-fat ratio.
- Improves the skin texture.
- Increases the metabolic rate.
- Increases muscle strength.

### Suggested Dose

Follow the manufacturer's guidelines.

### Note

HGH therapy is very expensive, costing $1,000 to $3,000 per month. It should be monitored by a qualified health professional.

Several natural products and practices stimulate HGH release from the pituitary gland. They include:

- Androstenedione
- Branched-chain amino acids
- Colostrum
- Exercise
- Glutamine
- L-arginine
- L-lysine
- L-ornithine
- L-tyrosine
- Oral HGH homeopathic sprays
- Weight training

## Melatonin

Melatonin is secreted by the pineal gland. The pineal gland is called the "regulator of the regulators." It is responsible for modulating the daily and the seasonal hormone levels. Melatonin is the hormone researchers now know regulates the body's biological clock. Used extensively as a sleep aid, it is also very popular for relieving the symptoms of jet lag, due to its ability to reset the body's internal clock. Researchers have found that melatonin also increases endorphin activity, which heightens the sensory feelings associated with sexual coitus. It also reduces the cholesterol levels, which prevents hardening of the arteries, thus staving off impotency. Furthermore, melatonin helps stabilize the thyroid function, thereby affecting the energy levels and body temperature, while promoting a feeling of well-being.

### Additional Benefits

- Prevents atrophy of the sexual organs.
- Boosts immunity.
- Relieves stress.
- Has antiaging capabilities.
- Fights depression.
- Has antioxidant capabilities.

### Suggested Dose
Take 1 to 3 milligrams at bedtime for sleep on an as-need basis.

### Note
To maintain or restore youthful melatonin levels, Dr. Walter Pierpaoli, William Regelson, and C. Coleman, authors of *The Melatonin Miracle* (Simon & Schuster, 1995), recommend the following dosages, all to be taken daily at bedtime:

For ages 40 to 45, .5 to 1 milligram
For ages 45 to 54, 1 to 2 milligrams
For ages 55 to 64, 2 to 2.5 milligrams
For ages 65 to 74, 2.5 to 5 milligrams
For ages 65 to 75, 2.5 to 5 milligrams
For ages 75 and older, 3.5 to 5 milligrams

## Pheromones

Part of what makes the sexual experience extremely pleasurable and exciting is the heightened awareness of our senses. An important sense sexually is the sense of smell. All people emit certain odors and subliminal scents. These scents are part of what attracts us to one another and in many cases determine with whom we mate and copulate. These scents, scientifically known as pheromones, have spawned a whole array of products, from sprays, fragrances, and body oils, to additives that are put in lotions, colognes, and perfumes.

According to research on the mating habits of animals, an organ is found in most vertebrate animals that serves as the mechanism for detecting certain chemical odors that are essentially undetectable. The organ is called the vomeronasal organ (VNO). In rats, the VNO is a small pair of sacs found on the vomer bone behind the nostrils, according to Neeraja Sankaran in her article, "The Science of Sex: What Is It and Who's Doing It?," published in *The Scientist* in 1999. Mrs. Sankaran adds that standard anatomy texts state that the VNO in humans dissipates during embryonic development.

However, current research by Charles Wysocki of the Monell Chemical Senses Center in Philadelphia shows that the VNO in humans also consists of two sacs. The sacs open into two shallow pits on each side of the nasal septum. Scientists now contend that the sensory cells that line these sacs are different from the olfactory cells found in the nose. It is in these sacs, researchers believe, that VNO detects the odors called pheromones.

Chemist Keith Slessor and biologist Mark Winston of British Columbia's Simon Fraser University, who won a gold medal in science and engineering from British Columbia for their research on honeybee queen pheromones, call pheromones our chemical calling cards. They are liquids produced by specialized cells or glands that don't necessarily elicit lust but serve to attract the opposite sex. In fact, Alan Hirsch, neurological director at the Smell and Taste Treatment Foundation in Chicago, has discovered in his research that individuals who lose their sense of smell many times lose their functional sexual capabilities. Psychologist Piet Vroon of the University of Utrecht in the Netherlands and author of *Smell: The Secret Seducer* (Farrar, Straus and Giroux, 1994) says that in many animal species, an intact olfactory organ is necessary for proper sexual behavior. Our sensory perceptions also affect the hypothalamus, which plays a role in the lubrication and swelling that occur during the course of the sexual excitement phase.

Agriculturists are now using the science behind pheromones to keep fruit flies from damaging crops in their $22 billion industry. The California Department of Food and Agriculture uses pheromones to trap male fruit flies before they can mate. This avoids the use of excessive amounts of pesticide.

While there is still considerable debate over whether pheromones actually work in humans, research is continuing into the efficacy of these natural agents. So far, it has been shown that in humans, an unidentified chemical component giving off a distinct odor that attracts members of the opposite sex is found in the glands at the base of hair follicles. These pheromones seem to best emit their scent from the armpits and the genital area.

Pheromones are marketed in the form of colognes, oils, and fragrances for both men and women. They are even available in products such as scented underwear.

### Additional Benefits
None.

### Suggested Dose
Follow the manufacturer's guidelines.

## Progesterone

Progesterone is another hormone found in women. It works with estrogen to regulate the menstrual cycle and to synchronize the many hormonal changes a woman experiences. It is released during the second half of the cycle and helps to prepare the uterus to accept and nurture the fertilized egg. If the released egg isn't fertilized, progesterone production begins to drop until the beginning of the next menstrual cycle. The uterine lining prepared for the egg degenerates and is eliminated via the menstrual flow.

Today, healthcare professionals know that replacing estrogen alone is very risky. They have found that by adding progesterone, the risk is greatly reduced. There are, however, problems associated with the use of progestin, the synthetic version of progesterone and the form usually used. These problems include:

- Breast tenderness
- Depression
- Weight gain

- Elevated cholesterol levels
- Abnormally heavy menstrual flow
- Fluid retention
- Migraine headaches

The natural forms of progesterone, the data clearly show, are safer than the synthetic forms and offer similar benefits. However, since some forms, such as the creams and gels, are not potent enough to offset the dominance of estrogen, they still need to be used with caution.

Despite the side effects, the use of progesterone along with estrogen has dramatically reduced the incidence of uterine cancer.

### Additional Benefits

- Relieves PMS symptoms.
- Controls the severity of hot flashes.
- Relieves insomnia.
- Reduces the episodes of painful periods.
- Controls excessive bleeding.
- Helps build bones.

### Suggested Dose

Follow your doctor's orders or the manufacturer's guidelines, depending on the particular product you use.

### Note

Some natural progesterones are extracted from peanut oil. If you are allergic to peanuts, please notify your healthcare provider.

## Testosterone

Testosterone is known as an androgen hormone and is found predominantly in males. Women also produce this hormone but in much smaller quantities. Like estrogen in women, testosterone is the hormone responsible for giving a male his masculine characteristics. It ebbs and flows at a torrid pace, always driving men's sexual thoughts and fantasies. Because of this fact, the sex drive in men, especially in younger men, is extremely high and intense.

As testosterone production diminishes over time, males begin to lose their sexual energy, drive, and vitality. This period of decline in males has been scientifically validated and is similar to what women experience at menopause. Health officials have dubbed this period male menopause, viropause, or andropause, all interchangeable terms. Marc Goldstein, M.D., a professor of urology at New York Hospital–Cornell Medical Center, reminds us that abnormally low levels of testosterone can occur at any age. In younger men, this condition is called hypogonadism.

Just as estrogen therapy contributes to a female's well-being, so does testosterone therapy help men. It can build lean muscle tissue, increase strength, improve sexual functioning, increase libido, stimulate HGH production, support immune function, and increase cognitive functions.

However, also like estrogen therapy, it has risk factors, including:

- Increased risk of cancer
- Atrophy of the testicles
- Depression
- Fluid retention
- Reduced sperm count
- High red blood cell and hematocrit count

Because of these risk factors, testosterone replacement should be administered by a qualified healthcare professional.

Testosterone is available in sublingual lozenges, injections, creams, gels, suppositories, and transdermal and glan patches.

### Additional Benefits

- Increases muscle size and strength.
- Decreases cholesterol levels.
- Prevents heart disease.
- Increases bone density.
- Has some correlation to the frequency of engaging in sexual intercourse.
- Heightens sexual arousal.
- Helps maintain erections.

### Suggested Dose
Follow your doctor's orders.

**Note**

Several natural products and practices produce results similar to those of testosterone but without the risks. They include:

- Consuming moderate amounts of fat and cholesterol
- Exercise
- Horny goat weed
- Soy isoflavens
- Stress reduction techniques
- Tribulus terrestis
- Vitamins A and D
- Weight training (especially bench pressing)
- Yohimbe
- Zinc

## Pregnenolone

Although not very well known, pregnenolone is considered to be the body's most basic hormone. Pregnenolone is manufactured from cholesterol and converted into progesterone. DHEA researchers maintain that a lack of production of pregnenolone could possibly slow down the manufacture of both estrogen and testosterone, thus directly affecting the sex drive. Like several other hormones, it starts to decline at about age 30, according to Ray Sahelian, M.D., author of *Pregnenolone: Nature's Feel Good Hormone* (Avery, 1997).

### Additional Benefits

- Alleviates depression.
- Enhances memory.
- Enhances sensory perception.
- Stimulates sex hormone production.
- Improves the auditory capabilities.
- Heightens immune cell activity.
- Normalizes the blood pressure.

### Suggested Dose

Take 5 to 10 milligrams daily.

*Note*

Dosages of 30 milligrams or more can cause insomnia, headaches, mood swings, and irritability.

## Vitamins and Minerals

Well-known naturopathic physicians such as Dr. Michael Murray have spent countless hours researching the effects that vitamin and mineral supplements have on human health. It has taken several decades, but the tide has changed in reference to the use of vitamin and mineral supplements as merely a way to make up for nutritional deficiencies. Scientists and healthcare professionals now realize that these substances are not only necessary to sustain life, but can be used to combat stress, boost immune function, and help the body recover from illness. Many of the country's most prestigious research facilities and institutions are backing this belief. Even prominent physicians such as Art Ulene, M.D., have retracted earlier negative verdicts on the use of vitamin and mineral supplements.

Dr. Ulene now boldly suggests that no matter how old you are, no matter the status of your health, new research shows that taking optimum dosages of the vitamins and minerals can improve your health. This revised opinion is shared by such notable health authorities as the late Nobel Prize–winning chemist Linus Pauling, Ph.D., Andrew Weil, M.D., Ronald Katz, M.D., Deepak Chopra, M.D., Joseph Pizzorno, N.D., and Earl Mindell, Ph.D., R.Ph. It was also discussed in an article in the *New England Journal of Medicine* in November 2001.

Evidence continues to mount concerning certain vitamins and minerals that help to moderate or regulate sexual function or desire. Many of these supplements also directly influence hormonal balance, acting as cofactors in the sexual communication system.

Here we will discuss the vitamin and mineral supplements that contribute to the maintenance, preservation, and enjoyment of sexual health.

### Vitamin A

Vitamin A is necessary for the proper production of the sex hormones and works to support adrenal function. It also plays a role in the manufacture of sperm, as well as in keeping the mucous tissue of the vagina in a youthful state.

### Additional Benefits

- Functions as a powerful antioxidant.
- Influences immunity.
- Essential to the health of the skin.
- Protects against cancer.
- Functions in vision.
- Encourages fertility.

### Suggested Dose

Take 5,000 to 10,000 international units daily.

### Note

Women who may become pregnant should not take more than 10,000 international units of vitamin A. If you are pregnant or lactating, consult your doctor.

## Vitamin B-Complex

The vitamin B-complex consists of eleven different B vitamins. Since they work synergistically, they all should be taken. Vitamins $B_1$, $B_6$, and $B_{12}$, niacin, and folic acid are well known. Vitamin $B_5$ (pantothenic acid), however, is very underrated. Found abundantly in the adrenal glands, vitamin $B_5$ assists the body in fighting stress. Overworked adrenals, as already discussed, cause a diminished sexual appetite. Many of the B vitamins are involved in testosterone production, sperm development, and pituitary gland function.

### Additional Benefits

See the individual B vitamins.

### Suggested Dose

Take 50 milligrams of a B-complex formula daily.

## Vitamin $B_3$

Vitamin $B_3$ (niacin) has gained national attention due to its ability to lower LDL cholesterol levels. Niacin dilates the blood vessels and heightens the bright red glow known as the sex flush. Sexual health researchers insist that niacin can increase the intensity and pleasurable feelings of an orgasm.

### Additional Benefits

- Breaks down fat, promoting arterial health.
- Decreases depression and irritability.
- Increases blood flow to the extremities.
- Improves circulation.
- Treats schizophrenia.

### Suggested Dose
Take 14 to 20 milligrams daily.

## Vitamin C

Vitamin C is sometimes called the master vitamin. Highly concentrated in the adrenal glands, it has powerful antioxidant capabilities. Antioxidants protect the system against free radicals. Free radical damage to the cells have been implicated in more than 60 age-related diseases. Free radicals are ever present and are formed as a result of normal metabolic activity. Poor lifestyle habits, environmental hazards, and smoking all increase free radical production. Vitamin C neutralizes free radicals. Essential for proper tissue growth and repair, and sperm production and motility, vitamin C also is critical to sex gland function and the sex drive.

### Additional Benefits

- Functions in the production of estrogen.
- Inhibits hardening of the arteries.
- Transports cholesterol from the arteries to the liver for processing.
- Protects the arterial walls from plaque buildup.
- Reduces the risk of cervical cancer.
- Eases the symptoms of oral herpes.

### Suggested Dose
Take 1,000 to 3,000 milligrams daily.

## Vitamin E

For years, vitamin E has been known as the sex vitamin and has been used to treat the problems associated with erectile dysfunction. Folklore aside, vitamin E assists in the transportation of oxygen in the blood. In both men and women this is critical to the proper functioning of the erectile tissue. Rich oxygenated blood facilitates proper erections and sensitivity, and preserves the youthfulness of the skin and tissues.

Vitamin E also helps relieve PMS symptoms and promotes normal blood clotting. It is crucial to proper circulation and dilation of the blood vessels. It also is a powerful antioxidant.

### Additional Benefits

- Relieves menopausal hot flashes.
- Combats aging.
- Prevents anemia and red blood cell destruction.
- Prevents testicular degeneration.
- Discourages the oxidation of polyunsaturated fats, thus strengthening the cell membranes.

### Suggested Dose

Take 200 to 800 international units daily.

## Folic Acid

Part of the B-vitamin family, folic acid has received much press over the last decade. Researchers now know it is responsible for protecting against neural tube birth defects. Therefore, women of childbearing age are encouraged by the Centers for Disease Control in Atlanta, Georgia, to take up to 400 micrograms of folic acid daily. Folic acid also supports proper ovarian function.

### Additional Benefits

- Inhibits anemia.
- Encourages proper red blood cell formation.
- Prevents heart disease.
- Helps vitamin $B_{12}$ to break down amino acids.
- Alleviates depression and anxiety.

- Discourages cervical dysplasia (a precancerous condition of the cervix).

*Suggested Dose*
Take 400 to 800 micrograms daily.

## Chromium

Are you at risk for high cholesterol levels, obesity, or blood sugar abnormalities such as diabetes or hypoglycemia? Chromium is used by millions of Americans to curb appetite, control blood sugar, and burn body fat. It can indirectly preserve your sexual health by contributing to your overall well-being and reducing the risk factors just mentioned.

*Additional Benefits*

- Facilitates protein synthesis.
- Increases the liver uptake of cholesterol and fatty acids.
- Improves the ratio of HDLs to LDLs.
- Prevents atherosclerosis.
- Controls mood swings.

*Suggested Dose*
Take 800 micrograms daily.

## Magnesium

Magnesium recently gained worldwide attention due to its ability to combat the negative effects of chronic fatigue syndrome. It is essential for proper nerve transmission and muscle function, which are important to sensory perception, touching, and foreplay. In addition, it has some specific benefits for women, as it helps alleviate PMS symptoms due to its role in progesterone production. Magnesium also assists in the manufacture of other hormones.

*Additional Benefits*

- Encourages elimination.
- Regulates the pH balance.
- Functions in energy production.

- Directly affects the electrical and physical actions of the heart muscle.
- Controls the blood pressure.
- Elevates the mood.

### Suggested Dose
Take 700 milligrams daily.

## Selenium

Selenium, considered a toxic element until a few years ago, is now one of the most sought-after supplemental minerals. This is due in part to its ability to combat and prevent cancer cell proliferation, especially in the prostate and breast. In males selenium is highly concentrated in the testes, and during ejaculation, selenium stores can reach fairly low levels. Because of this, researchers suggest that males supplement their diet with selenium. Women, too, should take supplemental selenium, since the American soil, and thus the food supply, is severely depleted of this mineral. Selenium also promotes progesterone production.

### Additional Benefits

- Improves mental alertness.
- Counteracts muscular weakness.
- Works synergistically with vitamin E.
- Keeps tissue pliable and elastic.
- Functions in the reproduction process.

### Suggested Dose
Take 200 micrograms daily.

## Zinc

Zinc is commonly called the sexy mineral. Without zinc, the sex organs cannot mature. In males, the mineral is concentrated in the prostate gland and promotes good prostate health. It also prevents the testes from shrinking, which can occur due to insufficient blood supply, infection, chemotherapy or radiation therapy, or malnutrition. Anecdotal evidence indicates that oysters have strong aphrodisiac properties and improve sexual functioning. According to Dr. Arnold Pike, author of *Nutrition Benefits of Oyster Extract* (Sagawa Publishers, 1980), this is due to their high zinc content. Zinc is also beneficial to proper immune function.

### Additional Benefits

- Responsible for the activation and function of more than 90 zinc-dependent enzyme systems.
- Improves thymus gland function.
- Strengthens the arteries.
- Promotes wound healing.
- Prevents impotency.

### Suggested Dose
Take 50 milligrams daily.

# Whole Green Foods and Phytochemicals

Research has revealed the existence of an arsenal of natural chemical components that are just as powerful as, if not more powerful than, vitamins and minerals. These components are found in whole foods, primarily fruits and vegetables, and are called phytonutrients. While the terminology surrounding these natural chemical components is still in flux, the nutrients themselves are known to protect not only general well-being, but also long-term health.

A particular class of foods that is rich in phytonutrients is whole green foods. Whole green foods are deep green leafy vegetables that have high concentrations of enzymes, including the digestive enzymes, and minerals such as calcium, potassium, and the trace minerals. In addition, they have heavy concentrations of chlorophyll, which helps to oxygenate the body, and are excellent tools for balancing the body's pH by raising its alkalinity.

In the following pages, we will discuss six phytonutrients that can play strong roles in your sexual health regime.

## Bee Pollen

Often called nature's most complete food, bee pollen contains every nutrient needed to create new living cells. Packed with an abundant supply of enzymes, amino acids, trace elements, and vitamins, especially the B vitamins, it also contains linoleic and linolenic acids, two key fatty acids that cannot be made by the body and must be supplied through the diet. Research conducted by Remy Chauvin, M.D., and colleagues at the Institute of Bee Culture in Bures Sur Yvete, France, has validated the traditional uses of bee pollen, including:

- To serve as a natural antibiotic.
- To regulate the intestinal flora.
- To combat allergy symptoms.
- To boost the immune response.
- To fight the effects of chronic fatigue.

More important to sexual health, bee pollen plays a role in the release of adenosine triphosphate (ATP), the high-energy compound that runs our system. ATP directly affects our sexual vitality, nourishes our reproductive system, and reenergizes our cells to carry out life's processes.

### Additional Benefits

- Balances the hormonal systems.
- Fights depression.
- Combats stress.

### Suggested Dose

Follow the manufacturer's guidelines. Bee pollen works best when taken on an empty stomach 15 to 20 minutes prior to physical activity.

## Chlorophyll

When you need to recharge your batteries, boost your energy levels, or detox you system, consider supplementing your diet with this "super-food." Chlorophyll is the green pigment that plants use to capture the power-packed rays of the sun. Humans convert chlorophyll into ATP, the energy that runs our bodies. This is because chlorophyll's molecular structure is similar to that of our blood. By revitalizing your cells' energy capacity, you can keep your system primed and energized for any sexual encounter. Chlorophyll also assists the body in reducing its toxic load, thus preserving not only sexual health, but also general well-being.

### Additional Benefits

- Promotes oxygenation of the body tissues.
- Builds red blood cells.
- Purifies the blood.
- Has antimutagenic potential.
- Counteracts upper respiratory tract infections.

### Suggested Dose
Follow the manufacturer's guidelines.

## Grape Seed Extract

Grape seed extract is one of the most powerful antioxidants known to humankind. Fifty times stronger than vitamin C or E in its antioxidant capabilities, it is considered one of the most potent preventative medicines you can take. Grape seeds are rich in a bioflavonoid compound complex called procyanidolic oligomers (PCOs). These bioflavonoid agents strengthen the arteries, veins, and connective tissue throughout the human body. They also protect the tissue from free radical damage, and keep the tissue—especially the blood vessels and joints—youthful and pliable. In addition, they ensure proper blood flow, thus improving sexual performance and keeping the sexual organs in good shape.

### Additional Benefits

- Has anti-inflammatory properties.
- Inhibits hardening of the arteries.
- Protects against cataract formation and glaucoma.
- Acts as a natural antihistamine.
- Combats the complications associated with asthma and emphysema.

### Suggested Dose
Take 1 milligram daily for every 1 pound of body weight for one week (to saturate the body tissues). Then take half that dosage daily there-

after, according to Clark Hansen, M.D., founder of the Southwest College of Naturopathic Medicine and Health Sciences in Scottsdale, Arizona.

### Note
PCOs are also found in blueberries, bilberries, pine bark, cranberries, and hazel nut tree leaves, but the highest concentration is found in grape seeds.

"Proanthocyanidin" and "procyanidolic oligomers" are names for the bioflavonoids found in grape seed extract.

## Noni

A tropical Hawaiian fruit, noni recently gained national attention due to its varied restorative, healing, and preventive health properties. Research out of the University of California at Los Angeles, the University of Hawaii, and Union College in London, England, has confirmed its multiple health-giving benefits. These include:

- Regulating the blood pressure.
- Modulating pain.
- Increasing alertness and energy levels.
- Improving sexual performance.
- Stimulating T-cell production.
- Controlling high blood pressure.
- Normalizing blood sugar levels.

According to botanist Dr. Isabelle Abbott, noni contains a powerful nutrient called scopoletin. This phytonutrient has shown the ability to dilate previously constricted blood vessels, increasing the circulation to the heart and other arteries, including the penile and pelvic arteries. Furthermore, evidence indicates that noni plays a major role in modulating the pineal gland, which regulates the activity of melatonin and serotonin, hormones connected with mood and sexual vitality.

### Additional Benefits
None.

### Suggested Dose
Take 2 ounces a half hour before breakfast and a half hour after dinner.

## Oolong Tea

Known as the "black dragon," oolong tea has been used for centuries in Japan and in the Fujian Province of China, where history cites its first use some 400 years ago. Analysis of oolong tea has shown that it contains large quantities of polyphenols, tannins, and catechins. All these substances contribute to health via their antioxidant capabilities. In addition, daily consumption of oolong tea stimulates superoxide dismutase (SOD) activity. SOD is an enzyme that fuels the antioxidant system. Japanese researchers have discovered that oolong tea consumed three times daily, along with conventional medical treatments, improved recalcitrant atopic dermatitis, which causes skin lesions, as reported in the *Archives of Dermatology* in 2001.

### Additional Benefits

- Rejuvenates weak spleen and kidney function.
- Reduces dark spots on and wrinkling of the skin.
- Enhances immunity.
- Increases enzyme activity.
- Discourages elevation of the tryglyceride levels.
- Increases the metabolism, thus preventing obesity.

### Suggested Dose

Drink 1 cup of prepared tea daily.

## Sun Chlorella

Susan Smith Jones, Ph.D., fitness and health sciences practitioner, maintains that chlorella is the richest source of chlorophyll found on the earth. Sun chlorella, according to Dr. Jones, is a single cell plant that actually increases in size as it matures and manufactures its own food. This is in contrast to increasing in size by adding new cells, as most other plants do. Because it can normalize the body chemistry, chlorella is touted for its ability to promote a high level of wellness.

In essence, sun chlorella has the ability to recharge the sexual batteries and to help the body maintain homeostatis. When you supplement your diet with sun chlorella, you take in the components your body uses to repair its DNA and flood your system with the enzymes and nucleic acids it uses to repair and maintain its life processes. Scientists consider chlorella to be one of the richest food sources on earth. Containing more than 20 different vitamins and minerals, a good balance of amino acids, more vitamin $B_{12}$ than beef liver, and a vast array of trace minerals, it is known as a superfood. Furthermore, it has powerful antioxidant capabilities, which further guard your health and sexuality.

### Additional Benefits

- Detoxifies the system.
- Helps burn fat, thus controlling unwanted pounds.
- Improves memory and mental alertness.
- Combats aging.
- Lubricates the joints and skin.

### Suggested Dose
Follow the manufacturer's guidelines.

# 11

# Detoxify to Satisfy

*Aging is the effect of an energy flow on matter over time. It is inevitable, it is said that time heals all wounds. But time leads to the gradual accumulation of waste products that eventually wears out the body, even in the absence of disease.*

Jed Diamond
*Male Menopause* (Source Books, 1997)

Despite what we know about the process of aging, we should not take what Jed Diamond says too lightly. The process he describes above may possibly be the most important factor you need to consider in your efforts to regain or improve your sexual health. Modern-day natural healthcare practitioners have confirmed what ancient healers have known for centuries. Disease according to nonconventional practitioners is not directly caused by microbes or foreign agents. We coexist with good and bad bacteria all the time, for example. It is when the body becomes weakened and loses its ability to defend itself that disease takes over. Disease is the body's way of letting us know that something is wrong or out of sync. There is now a growing consensus among alternative and complementary healthcare professionals that this underresearched area of human health may be the biggest threat to humankind.

Our present-day lifestyle and the increase in the number of individuals suffering from degenerative diseases, including sexual dysfunction, are intimately connected. If you add up all the insults the body has to deal with today—such as stress, chemicals, food pollution, water pollution, and legal and illicit drugs—you will see that even a well-conditioned body can be affected. Dr. Sherry Rogers says that an "increase in the number of foreign chemicals called 'xenobiotics' can be found today in our building materials, furniture, appliances and even our carpets." According to current estimates, more than 20,000 chemicals and food additives have been developed in the last several decades. The problem with many of these foreign elements is that they mimic the actions of nutrients and hormones, but have a different effect than the nutrient or hormone on the target cell, organ, or process.

When you do the math, it is not difficult to see how such a delicate and precise communication system as your sexual system can become damaged. Factor in the normal aging process, poor nutritional habits, and lack of exercise, and you and your sexuality may be candidates for early retirement. Past advocates of noninvasive medical treatments like John H. Tilden, M.D., insisted that autointoxication is the cause of the deterioration of human health. Dr. Tilden in 1890 formulated the Retentional Theory of Disease Causation. According to Dr. Tilden, when nerve energy is dissipated for any cause—physical disorders, mental problems, or bad habits—the body becomes enervated (deprived of nerve force, strength, or energy). He said that "when enervated, elimination is checked, causing retention of toxins within the blood and tissues we call toxemia."

The late Bernard Jensen, Ph.D., author of *Dr. Jensen's Guide to Better Bowel Care* (Avery, 1998), also insisted that autointoxication is the number one source of much of the misery and health decay we are witnessing in our society today. He said that it is much easier to avoid this toxic state in your youth than to have to struggle with the consequences in your later life. Other experts like Dr. Rogers refer to this problem as the body's "toxic waste load."

## Sex, Diet, and the Toxic Load

As already mentioned, one contributor to our toxemia is our highly processed food supply. Dr. Rogers in her research has found that many of the body's enzyme systems can no longer operate properly because the nutrient cofactors they require are no longer available in our nutrient depleted food supply. She says that many of the chemicals we get instead can even cause changes in the genetic material of our cells that can lead to cancer. When you really analyze Dr. Tilden's retentional theory of disease, Dr. Jensen's theory of autointoxication, and Dr. Rogers's theory of toxic overload, you see that it is short of miraculous that more of us are not sexually dysfunctional. The unhealthier, the more unstable, and the more weakened our internal body systems become, the more health problems and sexual problems we suffer from as a species.

This situation was discussed by Burton Goldberg in an article, "What We Must Do to Survive the 21st Century," in the January 2000 issue of *Alternative Medicine Digest*. In the article, Goldberg made note of the increasing number of children born with birth defects as well as the alarming number of infertile individuals in the United States. As these numbers continue to escalate, Goldberg cautioned, our ability to reproduce ourselves is becoming compromised.

In this chapter, we will discuss detoxification and internal cleansing. We will learn how to discourage the enervated stagnation of which Dr. Tilden spoke and will review how to naturally manipulate the actions of our internal systems to ensure that we remain in perfect sexual health.

Unless otherwise noted, the protocols discussed in this chapter are for both sexes, are inexpensive and safe, and can be done in the privacy of your own home. If you prefer professional assistance, ask your healthcare provider for a recommendation. Many of the programs outlined here can be done without professional help, however, and require just a small amount of your time. Most can be easily incorporated into your current schedule or daily routine.

The key according to Cheryl Townsley, author of *Cleansing Made Simple* (LFH Publishing, 1997), is not to be overwhelmed by the variety of cleansing programs. The best thing to do, she says, is to identify one or two protocols that you can successfully and consistently implement. "The easier the cleanse," she says, "the easier for you and the more your confidence is built."

## Chelation Therapy

Chelation therapy is a noninvasive process used to clean heavy metals and calcium deposits from arteries and veins. It consists of intravenous infusion of an amino acid using a small, 25-gauge needle. The therapy was pioneered by Elmer M. Cranton, M.D., author of *Bypassing Bypass* (Medex Publishers, 1997).

Chelation therapy is controversial but is gaining acceptance as a viable alternative to dangerous surgery and drugs for treating problems associated with clogged arterial pathways. As you know, clogged arteries can lead to strokes and heart disease, necessitating bypass surgery, balloon angioplasty, and other invasive procedures. The problem with these conventional procedures is that they target only certain blood vessels. Many patients after having these procedures need to go under the knife again several years later due to reclogging in the same artery or development of new clogs in additional arteries. There is a growing consensus that a whole body approach would better serve the patient than cardiovascular surgery, since surgery does nothing to stop or reverse the underlying cause of a disease.

Researchers have found that chelation therapy cleans out clogged arteries and blood vessels safely and effectively. Dr. Michael Gerber, past president of the Orthomolecular Medical Society, maintains that chelation therapy also restores lost vigor to depressed sexual organs by clearing clogged arteries and veins.

Dr. Gerber, a member of the American College of Advancement in Medicine and a diplomate in chelation therapy since 1984, says that chelating sessions can last from one to three hours. The chelating solution contains ethylene-diamine-tetraacetic acid (EDTA), as well as amino acids, minerals, and other natural chelating agents. Dr. Gerber says that "along with the infusion of chelating agents, nutrients like magnesium chloride, ascorbic acid (vitamin C), vitamin $B_{12}$, and B-complex are in some cases also introduced." During a treatment, the patient is seated in a comfortable chair or recliner, and can read, watch television, or take a nap. Depending upon the severity of the diseased arteries or the illness, the treatments are administered from once every other month to one to three times a week. Researchers have found that the EDTA solution does not react with other body chemicals or break down beneficial substances.

Chelation treatments should be administered by a licensed medical or alternative practitioner who has successfully completed oral and written exams given by the American Board of Chelation Therapy (ABCT). The side effects of chelation therapy are usually mild and include irritation at the infusion site, dizziness, headaches, nausea, and skin reactions. More serious side effects include decreased clotting ability, anemia, insulin shock, and kidney dysfunction. Before having a procedure, you should have a full workup including medical history done by a qualified healthcare professional. To find a qualified chelation practitioner in your area, contact the American College of Advancement in Medicine in Laguna Hills, California, at 714-583-7666.

For information on nonintravenous methods of chelation therapy through the use of over-the-counter oral chelating agents, see *The Chelation Way* by Dr. Morton Walker (Avery, 1990).

## Colon Cleansing

Colon cleansing is exactly what the name implies—cleansing of the large intestine of the gastrointestinal tract. Also called a high colonic, colon cleansing is accomplished by inserting a tube into the rectum and flushing the large intestine with about 20 gallons of water using a special machine. The water cleans away any waste materials that may be adhering to the walls of the colon.

The colon can be compared to a garbage disposal sewage system. It is responsible for reducing the harmful effects of waste by-products and for eliminating the waste from the body. It is also responsible for the absorption of fluids and electrolytes into the body. Electrolytes are dissolved minerals that supply the electrical power that keeps our system charged and in good working order. For this reason electrolytes are called the sparks of life.

Today researchers believe that waste by-products accumulate on the lining of the colon, causing it to become impacted. This can result in fatigue, decreased metabolic efficiency, digestive inefficiency, and proliferation of harmful bacteria. Many of these toxic by-products can also weaken the lining of the colon, making their way into the bloodstream, where they can then depress the central nervous system function, cause allergic reactions, and weaken the immune system. This weakening of the lining of the colon is known as leaky gut syndrome.

Leaky gut syndrome can be compared to a slow leak in an automobile tire. Under normal conditions, the mucous lining of the colon allows beneficial nutrients and digested foods to pass into the bloodstream. When the lining is compromised, it also allows unwanted food particles, waste, and toxic materials to enter the system and wreak havoc. One complication that can result is activation of the body's autoimmune response system. Here, the body attacks its own tissues, since it perceives them as foreign invaders. In the long run, this can affect your well-being and your sexuality.

To keep your colon clean, healthy, and efficient, have a high colonic periodically, once or twice a year. To find a qualified therapist, ask your healthcare practitioner for a referral.

There are now also many colonic systems that can be used at home. Seek professional help until you become adept in their use. Individuals suffering from heart disease and other chronic conditions should check with their healthcare providers before undergoing any kind of colonic treatment.

In addition to having regular high colonics, keep your colon clean by consuming 25 to 50 grams of fiber daily. Supplement your diet daily with beneficial bacterial such as: bifidobacterium, lactobacillus acidophilus, and lactobacillus bulgaricus. Available in tablet and liquid form, these bacteria will help keep pathogenic bacteria at bay, rendering them harmless. These friendly bacteria will also help prevent or treat vaginitis, urethritis, and cystitis, disorders that can put a damper on even the healthiest sex drive.

Take a fructooligosaccharides supplement daily. Commonly known as FOS, it acts as fast food for friendly bacteria. FOS actually helps friendly bacteria stay healthy and multiply.

Consume generous helpings of complex carbohydrates daily. Acidophilus bacteria actually feed off carbohydrates and lactose (milk sugar). Red meat discourages good colon health.

Finally, consume eight to ten glasses of water daily. This will flush your kidneys of impurities and help the fiber you consume work more effectively.

## Detox Baths

Water is the great healer. To jump-start sluggish or toxin-laden sexual organs, consider the power of water. Detox baths are great for relieving stress and bringing you back to your sexual self. They are also excellent for increasing the circulation and blood flow, and opening up the pores of the skin to facilitate the removal of internal toxins.

There are many variations of detox baths. One is the Epsom salt bath. About two to three times a week, do the following:

1. Fill your bathtub with water as hot as you can tolerate.
2. Mix about ¼ to ½ cup of Epsom salts into the bath water.
3. Immerse yourself in the water and soak until the water becomes lukewarm.
4. Do not towel dry yourself. Instead, wrap yourself in a cotton bathrobe and lie down until you are dry.
5. Take a warm shower, then head straight for bed. (Before going to bed, drink at least 8 ounces of water.)

A detox bath can also be prepared using raw apple cider vinegar, baking soda, or equal parts of Epsom salts and baking soda. The whole process can be done one hour before bedtime. You will find that while you feel revitalized, you will also feel free of stress and anxiety, and will sleep very comfortably.

## Kidney and Bladder Cleansing

What do the kidneys and bladder have to do with sexual functioning? Indirectly quite a bit. The kidneys are a primary detoxification site. They filter your blood of waste and help you maintain a proper pH balance. The filtered waste by-products are excreted as urine through the urethra when your bladder is full. Individuals, particularly females, who suffer from recurring bladder and yeast infections know that these painful and annoying disorders can turn off even the most ferocious sexual appetite.

To keep the kidneys and bladder running smoothly, drink 8 to 10 glasses of fresh clean water every day to assist them in flushing out toxins. Do not become dehydrated. Drink a glass of water even before your body signals that you're thirsty.

Doctors use what is called a specific gravity test to ascertain the amount of pure water versus by-products contained in the urine. Too much sediment means the kidneys are not eliminating or neutralizing waste properly. This can lead to uric acid or kidney stone formation. These painful disorders will quickly send your sex drive south of the border. Alcohol, hot spices, peppers, mustard, and even excessive tea and coffee can also irritate the kidneys.

## Liver Cleansing

The liver is our internal miracle worker. Weighing only about 5 pounds, it is our lifeline to general health and sexual health. Without the powerful feats the liver performs, not only would your sexual health be compromised, but you could die. The liver detoxifies the blood and acts as a storage site for carbohydrates, vitamins, and minerals. It breaks down proteins, fats, and carbohydrates, and is responsible for bile formation. Bile is the liquid that is sent to the gallbladder to help metabolize fat properly. Without bile, your ability to maintain proper cholesterol levels would be hampered considerably.

Every minute of the day some 10 million red blood cells die and must be disposed of. The liver acts much like a recycling plant, detoxing these dead red blood cells, then using them to build new ones. Think of your liver as your poison control center. Everything you ingest, be it food, alcohol, prescription medicine, or caffeine goes to the liver to be broken down and rendered harmless. This prohibits toxic by-products from accumulating in the blood at dangerous or lethal levels.

When you do not take care of yourself and subject your normal avenues of elimination to toxic waste overload, you damage your sexual potential. If your liver, kidneys, colon, and other elimination sites become clogged, your body must find alternative dump sites. For example, in the case of a male with a toxic liver, the prostate gland can become an alternative dumping site, called an organ of "vicarious elimination" according to Dr. Henry Bieler in his book *Dr. Bieler's Natural Way to Sexual Health* (Charles Publishing, 1972). Any male who has suffered from prostatis (inflamed prostate gland) or an infection related to bacterial contaminants knows the intense pain that can occur with ejaculation. However, sexual inactivity to avoid the pain can lead to stagnation of the prostate fluid in the gland. Pain or sexual inactivity—neither choice is good.

One way to protect your liver is to drink generous amounts of sugar-free cranberry juice. Cranberry juice removes purines, which are uric acid by-products, from the bladder, kidneys, testicles, and prostate gland. Cranberry juice also inhibits bacteria's ability to attach to the walls of the bladder, thus discouraging urinary tract infections.

Another way to flush toxins from the liver is the liver-gallbladder flush. Once a month, at bedtime, drink 4 ounces of warm olive oil, followed by 4 ounces of orange or lemon juice. Go directly to bed and lie on your right side with your right knee pulled up to your chest for 30 minutes before going to sleep. The olive oil will induce contractions of the gallbladder, causing bile to be released, as well as bicarbonate and digestive enzymes to be expelled. This will help your system to maintain a good pH balance and to properly break down toxic by-products. It will also enhance your metabolism of fats and cholesterol.

In between your monthly liver-gallbladder flushes, do daily maintenance flushes. Simply mix 1 teaspoon of olive oil into 4 ounces of lemon, grapefruit, or orange juice, and drink. Do this when you first wake up, before you eat breakfast.

## pH Balance

The old saying that beauty is only skin deep is most appropriate when focusing on the preservation of your sexual health. As we have already discussed, pH balance is a silent but important component of general as well as sexual well-being. Imbalances in pH not only compromise your long-term health, but over time can interfere with the proper functioning of your sexual apparatus. Neither your cells nor your internal organs can operate very well in an acidic environment.

To test your pH levels at home, purchase a pH strip kit from your local health food store or pharmacy. The first thing in the morning, urinate into a clean plastic cup.

Dip a pH test strip in the urine, and compare the color of the strip with the color code that comes with the kit. Remember that on the pH scale, 8 to 14 means your system is too alkaline, encouraging the growth of harmful bacteria. This makes you more susceptible to yeast and urinary tract infections. If your reading is between 0 to 6 , your system is too acidic.

Your body can be compared to a beautiful home. Within the cracks and crevices of your home could be silent but malicious hoards of termites eating away at the foundation. This is the kind of internal bombardment your health and sexuality take when your internal pH goes awry.

**SPECIAL NOTE**

If you test your pH balance first thing in the morning and find that your reading shows you are alkaline, you actually may be too acidic. Your body during sleep actually produces bicarbonate to compensate for the state of disequilibrium and the threat to your health. Bicarbonate neutralizes excess acid. The body seeks to maintain a slightly alkaline pH level between 7.36 and 7.44. When your system remains in a highly acidic state, a little bit of your health and sexuality deteriorate each and every day.

To restore the balance if your system is too acidic:

- Eat more fresh fruits and vegetables.
- Reduce or eliminate soft drinks.
- Drink alkaline water every day.

You can make alkaline water by adding a few drops of ionized water and electrolytes to your regular water. Ionized water is rich in minerals that are electrically charged and well absorbed by the body. You can purchase small containers of ionized water at your local health food store.

The minerals obtained from fresh fruits and vegetables are added to a reserve of these electrically charged minerals in our tissues. The standard American diet, generally devoid of whole foods, is a major culprit in disrupting normal pH. Alkaline drops are an inexpensive way to boost your diet.

## Proper Rest

Proper rest is vital to the body's natural cleansing abilities and to proper immune system function. According to Cheryl Townsley, author of *Cleansing Made Simple* (LFH Publishing, 1997), the detoxification or cleansing process in adults is the major molecule-making activity performed by the body. It is when you are sleeping that most of your repair work and cleansing takes place. According to Ms. Townsley, the majority of the cleansing activity occurs between the hours of 1:00 A.M. and 3:00 A.M.

Internal cleansing requires an enormous amount of energy and is so vital that your body will delegate up to 80 percent of its energy pool toward that goal. Without proper rest, you will invariably increase your stress levels, overwork your adrenal glands, and compromise your ability to perform at your peak levels sexually. Get at least a solid 8 hours of sleep every night.

## Skin Brushing

One of the oldest methods of noninvasive internal cleansing is skin brushing. As the name implies, you actually brush your skin. The skin helps get rid of more waste by-products (especially cellular waste) than both the kidneys and liver combined. Skin brushing stimulates proper blood flow, as well as lymph flow. Lymph is the fluid that bathes the immune system. It picks up and drops off waste at dump sites known as lymph nodes. The lymph, however, is not pumped through the system like blood. To move, it requires help via exercise. Skin brushing also helps to move it through the system.

Skin brushing can be done with a medium- to firm-bristle brush. To do a skin brush, use gentle, circular motions over the entire body.

Brush your skin in the morning before you shower and again in the evening. Brush for about 5 to 10 minutes each session.

## Other Detox Methods

Periodic fasting, steam baths, saunas, mineral baths, massage therapy, and deep breathing techniques are additional ways to safely and naturally cleanse the body. Exercise, the forgotten hero, is also vital to reducing stress and cleansing the lymph system. Enzyme therapy, which assists proper nutrient breakdown and metabolism, is part of proper bowel management. These therapeutic methods of elimination are all cornerstones in the naturopathic tradition of cleansing, says Jill E. Stansbury, N.D., chairwoman of the Botanical Medicine Department of the National College of Naturopathic Medicine in Portland, Oregon. Dr. Stansbury insists that cleansing your body of old toxins is the first step to achieving radiant health. She also claims that it is a step too many people bypass.

To improve and preserve your overall health and sexual health, consider using herbs that are known for their cleansing abilities. Many of them can be taken orally, in tea form, as an infusion, or as liquid drops.

Some good herbs to consider are:

- Garlic, which cleanses the blood
- Milk thistle, which cleanses the liver
- Goldenseal, which purifies the blood
- Sarsaparilla, which cleanses the blood and lymph
- Ginger, which stimulates the circulation and encourages sweating
- Burdock root, which acts as a general cleanser

In addition, consuming energy-filled whole green foods such as wheat grass, chlorophyll, chlorella, and barley grass will go a long way in solidifying your efforts.

# 12

# Holistic Sex Secrets

*Developing your love making to the point where it is as plea-*
*surable and mutually satisfying as possible takes more than a*
*positive attitude, an erotic setting, or a specific technique. The*
*real secret is in developing sensuality—an appreciation for*
*the many nuances of feeling and the exquisite range of sensa-*
*tions of which the body is capable.*

Barbara Keesling, Ph.D.
*Sexual Pleasure* (Hunter House, 1993)

Mind/body pioneer Wilhelm Reich, M.D., who studied under Sigmund
Freud, maintained that many of our social ills as well as our diseases are
a direct result of the repression of our natural sexuality. According to an
article by Dr. Michael Gerber, "Reich and Role," published in the July
2000 issue of *Alternative Medicine Digest,* Dr. Reich developed a system
of sexual therapy called "character analysis." From this therapy he formulated a theory on the function of the orgasm. According to Dr. Reich,
the orgasm is not just a means for experiencing pleasure or creating new
life. He believed that the orgasm is also meant to reequilibrate the energy system of the entire body. This physical mechanism in Dr. Reich's
opinion is actually a natural method used by the body to improve and
maintain both physical and mental well-being.

Human beings, according to Dr. Reich, never really experience the
true nature and explosiveness of the orgasm due to our social condition-
ing. Dr. Reich believed that "total orgasm" can happen only when both

partners are completely free of what he referred to as "armor." This freeing oneself of armor is the same as Dr. Keesling's development of sensuality (see above). Lila Nachtigall, M.D., of the New York University School of Medicine, says that "in our society both men and women have been trained to believe that they lose their sex appeal over time." This false assumption causes many to repress their sexual feelings, fantasies, and intimacy. Developing sensuality, as well as generating health, requires a holistic approach, free of the armor Dr. Reich describes.

Chapter 12 is a compendium of ideas to restore, jump-start, rekindle, or preserve your sexual proficiency. These protocols more importantly are drug-free and in most cases will contribute to your body's efforts to remain strong, disease-free, and sexually active. The key is to realize that your sexual expressions of love and intimacy have deep-seated emotional ties. How and why you express yourself sexually are a matter of personal choice. The various ways in which you express yourself and your proficiency at doing so are intimately connected to your overall health and well-being, however.

Many people, according to Alexandra Penney in *How to Make Love to a Man* (Dell, 1990), are nervous about accepting pleasure and are often not aware of their anxiety (or armor). Many people feel it's perfectly okay to give pleasure and to touch, she says, but they're inhibited or feel guilty about accepting what feel goods. If you really take the time to explore your erotic nature, you can enhance your orgasmic pleasure and enrich your life.

Remove your armor and enjoy your and your partner's sexuality!

## Learning About the Erotic Zones

- Sexual aids such as dildos and vibrators are excellent tools for exploring your own erotic zones. Use these devices to learn how you respond when certain areas of your body are touched.
- After sexual intercourse or sexual stimulation without an orgasm, the clitoris remains erect for several hours. Try oral or manual stimulation of the clitoris while the woman remains aroused to still bring on an orgasm.
- The perineum in both males and females is highly erotic and an excellent area to explore during oral stimulation.
- You can ask for what you want sexually in a nonverbal way.

Guiding your partner's actions via body language or during fore-play can heighten his or her awareness. It may also be perceived as less threatening or critical.

- Practice your foreplay techniques. Study after study reveals that women rate foreplay as more important than orgasm. They also say that it can intensify their orgasms.
- Learn patience. Women take longer to reach orgasm than men do.
- Just before ejaculation, pressing on the man's perineum may delay ejaculation without disrupting the pleasurable sensation of the orgasm.

## Enhancing Orgasmic Pleasure

- Fantasize, fantasize, and fantasize. Let your imagination go. Your partner will be the benefactor.
- Touch and stroke a woman's clitoris in a sensual manner often.
- Gently stroke the head of the penis. The head is much more sensitive to the touch than the shaft.
- Tell your partner how you feel and what your preferences are.
- When engaging in oral stimulation of the vagina, focus on the labia minor, which during the height of stimulation become bright red. Move your tongue back and forth in a rhythmic motion.
- Give your male partner a prostate massage. Insert a lubricated finger into his rectum and press it toward the front of his body. You will find a spot (the prostate gland) that feels like a small-sized lump about the size of a chestnut. Gently massaging this area is highly stimulating and can cause intense, dynamic, and forceful orgasms. It is believed that the G-spot in females and the prostate gland in males originate from the same embryonic tissue.
- Do your sexercises (see Chapter 14) daily. They will help increase the blood flow and the sensations in your genital area.
- As you and your partner age, you may find your sexual roles changing. Women often become more aggressive sexually as they grow older, while men find their sex drive beginning to wane. This is part of the natural order of things. Don't resist it; enjoy it!
- Both men and women are very sensitive to anal stimulation, says Debora Phillips, M.D., coauthor of *Sexual Confidence* (Houghton Mifflin, 1980). She says rubbing the anus with your finger or very

gently inserting your finger into the anus can be very pleasurable. If you feel comfortable with anal stimulation, *which is not for everyone,* you might find that it adds to the intensity of your orgasm, especially if it is done just before the orgasm.

- Both the female clitoris and male penis are highly sensitive to the touch. The head of the penis has many more sensory filled nerves than the shaft, while the main purpose of the clitoris, as mentioned in Chapter 2, is to serve both as a receptor and transformer of sexual stimuli. Therefore, both the clitoris and penis are prime targets for manual and oral stimulation. The oral stimulation of the penis is called fellatio, while the oral stimulation of the clitoris is called cunnilingus.
- The scrotum, like the penis, is an erogenous zone that is highly sensitive to touch. Mantak Chia and Douglas Abrams, in their book *The Multi-Orgasmic Man* (HarperCollins, 1997), claim that scrotal tugging can delay a male's ejaculation and prolong lovemaking. The scrotum, which houses the testes, must pull up close to the body to expel semen. Therefore, encircling the top of the scrotal sac with a thumb and forefinger and gently pulling down on it at the height of the orgasmic phase can delay ejaculation.
- One of the most successful techniques used by sex therapists to help men conquer ejaculation problems is called the stop and start method. First used in the 1950s by Dr. James Semans, the method involves stimulating the man to the point just before ejaculation, then removing the stimulation and actively preventing ejaculation. To prevent ejaculation, squeeze the end of the penis (just below the head) for approximately 30 seconds. Repeat starting and stopping ejaculation as many times as desired.

## Increasing Sexual Stamina and Vitality

- Wait two to three hours after eating to have sex. Large meals disrupt the circulation, as blood flow is diverted to the digestive system. Not only can this interfere with the sensory feeling in your genital area, but stomach cramps can result when blood is forced into those muscles.
- An hour or two before you expect to engage in sexual intercourse,

consume several 8-ounce glasses of water. This will greatly assist proper blood flow to your erectile tissue.

- Stay physically active. Remember that sex is a physical act requiring mobility, stamina, and flexibility. Vince Lombardi, the late legendary Green Bay Packers football coach, once said that fatigue makes cowards of us all. Lack of vitality and being out of shape will surely increase your chances of becoming a sexual casualty.
- Sleep is an important factor in maintaining a robust sexual appetite. According to the National Sleep Foundation, the amount of sleep people get may be directly related to the frequency with which they have sex. Our sleep patterns are linked to our biological rhythms. Among the things that can disrupt our biological rhythms are depression, fatigue, accelerated aging, disruptions in the menstrual cycle, depressed immune function, diminished growth hormone production, and tension and stress.
- An hour or so before sexual contact, try using a natural sex stimulant rather than a drug to increase your sexual prowess, stamina, and pleasure.
- Avoid alcohol. Contrary to popular belief, it is a central nervous system depressant. Over time, it will actually diminish sensory feelings, and in males, it can contribute to erectile dysfunction.
- Women who have had growth hormone therapy have reported a substantial increase in their sex drive, an increase in sexual pleasure, and more orgasms.
- Frequent sex will restore youthful vigor to your sexual organs.
- Men should not clinch their pubococcygeous (PC) muscle when having an erection. The PC muscle, also known as the pelvic floor muscle, is the muscle both men and women use when urinating. Continued over a period of time, clenching this muscle will cause problems in the ability to maintain an erection. It prevents blood from flowing into the penile arteries.
- Studies show that the more sex men have, the higher their levels of testosterone will remain.
- Do not consume dairy products, especially milk, before a sexual encounter. Drinking a cup of hot milk before bed will relax you right to sleep.
- Consider a juice fast for 3 to 5 days when you want to build your sexual stamina. Drink organic, nonsweetened juice. Many natural

health practitioners report that short juice fasts substantially increase sexual vitality, appetite, and drive.

## Making Time for Whoopee

- If you have kids, designate one night out of the week as your night. Hang a DO NOT DISTURB sign on your door or hire a babysitter, and indulge in each other.
- When was the last time you took off for the weekend to smell the roses together? Whether you plan the weekend or take off on the spur of the moment is irrelevent. The important thing is to do it together.
- Be on constant alert for ways to restore intimacy to your relationship.
- Do not forget how to have fun with one another.

## Manipulating the Sexual Senses

- The skin is a bed of nerve endings that transmit sensory feeling. Rub on a bit of jasmine- or sandalwood-scented body lotion before a sexual encounter.
- Change your setting to prevent bedroom boredom. If you can't change the physical location of your setting, change the mood of your setting.
- Stop trying to be the perfect lover. Be creative and "go with the flow." Plan sexual getaways, and indulge in your fantasies.
- Prime yourself and your partner with an erotic massage.
- When having trouble reconnecting sexually after a period of emotional conflict, practice focal exercises. Take turns exploring and caressing each other's entire body for about 15 minutes. Do not have sexual intercourse, and do not bring each other to orgasm. Do this for a few weeks as a retraining exercise.
- Learn how to manipulate each other's sexual senses with exotic oils, perfumes, baths, and other aromatherapy techniques.

## Protecting Your Sexual Health

- Vaseline should not be used as a lubricant in anal or conventional sexual intercourse. It can dry out and weaken condoms. Better lubricants to use are K-Y Jelly and Astroglide.
- Women who have decided against hormone replacement therapy but are concerned about vaginal dryness, pain, and irritation should apply an estrogen cream to their labia, vagina, and vulva daily to restore moisture and prevent atrophy of the vaginal tissue.
- Avoid vaginal douches, since they indirectly help germs invade the vagina.
- Uncircumcised men should wash beneath the foreskin to avoid infections of the penile glans.
- If you smoke, quit. Cigarette smoking not only can cause cancer, emphysema, and other health problems, but is a major cause of erectile dysfunction. Smoking constricts the penile arteries. Dr. Ronald Katz suggests that giving up cigarettes to save your sex life may be a stronger motivator than to merely save your life.
- Take a liquid crystalloid mineral supplement daily to assist your body in restoring and maintaining proper pH balance and good blood flow to the pelvic and penile arteries.
- Weight training has some great effects on sexuality. Besides keeping the body toned, flexible, and strong, exercises such as leg squats and presses will help increase the blood flow to the penile arteries.
- Chronic bowel problems can negatively affect your sexual health. Keep your eliminative organs clean and free of toxic buildup.
- Tropical fruits such as pineapples, papayas, mangos, and bananas are loaded with natural enzymes that act like chelating agents, which break down plaque and cholesterol. Eat them often.
- Studies show that people who see themselves as sexual beings and as being desired actually live longer, recover from illness faster, and generally do better in other areas related to overall health and well-being.
- Nutrients such as vitamin E and coenzyme $Q_{10}$ ($CoQ_{10}$) help transport oxygen in the blood. Oxygen transportation is vital to maintaining sexual vitality.
- Practice deep breathing exercises. Good oxygenation, combined with nutritious food and clean fresh water, greatly assists cell re-

generation, balancing of the pH, production of the sex hormones, and maintenance of general and sexual well-being.

- Never allow yourself to believe that because you are aging you should expect a decline in your sexual wants and desires.
- Women should practice relaxing and contracting their vaginal muscles. This will keep the muscles strong and flexible.

## Adding Romance to Sex

- Bring home a dozen roses. Let your partner know that tonight is the night.
- Send a pair of your sexiest panties along with him to work in his briefcase.
- Have flowers delivered to her at her place of employment.
- Surprise your partner with some quality time for the two of you. Rearrange your schedule and take that trip you have been discussing.
- Relax and soak together in a hot tub of water with scented oils. Let nature take its course.
- Find something on which to compliment your partner. Switch roles for a day or a weekend. Learn to appreciate your partner's skills and the sacrifices he or she makes in the name of your relationship.

# PART V

# MANAGING YOUR SEXUAL POTENTIAL FOR LIFE

*Many people see sex as a source of shared joy. Others have come to view sex as an added source of stress, just one more area of life where they have to perform.*

*Perhaps the most insidious obstacle to sexual fulfillment is the image of the aging sex life. The myths persist despite studies showing that many couples are able to enjoy sex two to three times a week even when they're in their nineties. I suspect that many of us, trapped by misconception, never come close to realizing our lifelong potential for the sensory energy that we receive or express through sex.*

Robert K. Cooper, Ph.D.
*High Energy Living* (Rodale Press, 2000)

Our sexuality is a part of our wholeness, according to Robert K. Cooper, Ph.D., an independent health researcher and author of *High Energy Living* (Rodale Press, 2000). It is one of the ways our bodies use to maintain balance. How well our systems are able to neutralize the elements and forces that upset our equilibrium is vital to preserving our sexuality.

As we have already discussed, a body that is dysfunctional sexually is a body that is out of sync with the laws of nature. In Part V, we will take a look at stress, stressors, and stress energy, and how we adapt to them. Without a clear understanding of how sexual health is affected by stress, you will not be able to develop an effective plan to restore, maintain, or improve your sexual health. In addition, we will review why exercise is important to the preservation of your sexual health, why sexual inactivity is actually detrimental to preserving your sexual capabilities, and how to find help in preserving your sexual health and life-long potential. Health and sexuality are joined at the hip, so much so that Dr. Paul Pearsall, Ph.D., says in *A Healing Intimacy: The Power of Loving Connections* (Crown, 1995):

> Sexual fitness is so intrinsic to our general health that any doctor who ignores it practices bad medicine, and any person who forgets it, puts his or her entire well being at risk.

# 13

# Use It or Lose It

*Younger people can be heartened by the information that the more you use it, the less you lose it, which, is not true of any other bank account I've ever heard of.*

Mary S. Calderone, M.D., M.P.H.
*President, Sex Information and Education Council of the United States*

Atrophy is the wasting away of a body part. Is it possible for an individual's sexual organs to atrophy? The answer is yes. Both sexes are susceptible to this negative aspect of human sexuality due to a number of factors. Aging is one. Inactivity is another. In this chapter, we will discuss the effects of aging and inactivity, and how to combat them.

## Aging

Females begin to show signs of sexual atrophy as they approach menopause. As their estrogen levels decline, many women, according to Dr. David Reuben in *Everything You Always Wanted to Know About* Sex begin to lose interest in sex. According to Dr. Reuben, the vagina begins to shrivel, the uterus gets smaller, the breasts start to atrophy, and sexual desire begins to wane.

Dr. Lila E. Nachtigall paints a similar picture. She says that estrogen is responsible for the shape, size, and flexibility of the female vagina, and with the decreasing levels, the vaginal tissues become dryer, and the vagina becomes narrower, less pliable and expandable, and occasionally even a little shorter. She also says that in some cases the opening of the vagina atrophies to such an extent that intercourse can no longer occur.

Sexual health professionals now also know that as a woman's vaginal walls become thin and lose their ability to become lubricated, her susceptibility to vaginal infections increases. This is another major reason for women's diminished sexual desire and drive, as sexual intercourse can become very painful if not impossible.

## Inactivity

While estrogen is a cause of sexual-organ atrophy, there is also another reason, according to Joseph Poticha, M.D., author of *Use It or Lose It* (Richard Markek Publishers, 1978). The other cause, says Dr. Poticha, is lack of regular sexual stimulation. The above description of sexual atrophy is what Dr. Poticha means by "use it or lose it."

Sexual health researchers Masters and Johnson agree with Dr. Poticha. They found in their research that women who engage in regular sexual intercourse (at least once or twice a week) throughout the years preceding menopause remained more sexually active and anatomically in better shape after menopause. Regular sexual activity helps keep the mucosal secretions flowing, keeps the muscles of the vagina in good shape, and helps preserve the vagina's shape, size, and contour. Also agreeing is Robert Butler, M.D., former director of the National Institute on Aging and coauthor of *Love and Sex After 60* (Ballantine, 1993). Dr. Butler states that total abstinence from sexual contact for long periods of time can cause impotency problems in males and lubrication problems in women. Dr. Judith Reichman concurs with Dr. Butler. In fact, she says, one activity in which she insists her patients engage to preserve the youthfulness of their genitals is masturbation.

Many urologists who treat enlarged prostate glands prescribe sexual intercourse to their patients. As discussed in Chapter 1, the prostate is the small gland that is wrapped around the urethra. It manufactures the fluid that helps propel the semen through the urethra. The prostate gland is prone to bacterial infections, however, and when the other organs of elimination become congested, the prostate often becomes a dumping ground. Urologists argue that ejaculation discourages the stagnation of fluids and the buildup of toxins within the gland.

## Masturbation

Although sexual intercourse keeps the reproductive organs in good shape, it is not the only way. More and more healthcare professionals nowadays are saying that masturbation is a key factor in sexual health that should be practiced regularly. Dr. Nachtigall, in her research, found that women who regularly engage in masturbation or self-stimulatory techniques maintain more tone in their vaginal walls. Dr. Reuben says that masturbation is also extremely important for men. He claims that masturbation to orgasm actually keeps the body's physiological mechanisms in good working order. The body, according to Dr. Reuben, sees no difference between masturbation and sexual intercourse. Whether you masturbate or have intercourse, he says, your sexual communication system gets the workout it needs. Betty Dodson, in her book *Sex for One* (Harmony Books, 1987), calls masturbation an art form and our primary avenue of sexual expression.

Dr. Butler maintains that children often practice masturbation and that current thinking holds that self-stimulation in the early years is very important to the development of healthy adult sexuality. Studies on human sexuality done by experts such as Shere Hite, Dr. Alfred Kinsey, and Masters and Johnson all show that a high percentage (in some cases up to 80 percent and more) of American men and women engage in self-stimulation to reach orgasm. Dr. Butler states, "The evidence seems clear that although masturbation was once seen as a perversion and a cause of mental and physical disease, it is now recognized as a 'normal' sexual activity throughout life."

If this vital part of human sexuality causes you any emotional or psychological distress, you should consider talking to your healthcare professional and/or partner. To discover ways to enhance this experience, see Betty Dodson's book *Sex for One*.

When considering masturbation, it is important to remember the benefits that sexual health researchers have discovered concerning increased longevity in individuals who have an orgasm at least two times a week. Relieving stress and tension are added benefits.

*    *    *

Enjoying regular sexual activity will help preserve your sexual vitality. Abstinence is not always the best strategy for preserving sexual health. Use it, don't lose it, and enjoy yourself in the process.

In the next chapter, we will examine exercise's role in general and sexual health. Exercise is vital for maintaining the youthful state of your body, and exercising your genitals and pelvic area can actually heighten your sexual response and pleasure.

# 14

# What's Exercise Got to Do With It?

*Entropy or the second law of "thermodynamics" states that the amount or order in any system left to itself must eventually decrease until complete disorder results. In other words, sit on the sofa long enough, eating junk food and staring at the television, and you may disintegrate into a puddle of ugly cosmic goo.*

Daniel Mowrey, Ph.D.
"Get Moving," *Energy Times* (January 1996)

Unless you are Rip Van Winkle, you most likely have heard about all the findings concerning the health benefits of exercise. Most of what we now know about exercise physiology can be traced back to early studies conducted by Kenneth Cooper, M.D., founder and director of the Cooper Wellness Center, in Dallas, Texas. Today because of the efforts of Dr. Cooper and many other researchers, the health-giving benefits of regular exercise are common knowledge. However, even in our modern, high-tech society, the American sedentary lifestyle continues to be a problem.

It is, paradoxically, our fast-paced lifestyles, requiring convenience foods and labor-saving appliances, that health professionals claim are a major contributor to the rising incidence of degenerative diseases such as heart disease, diabetes, arthritis, hypertension, arteriosclerosis, osteoporosis, depression, chronic fatigue, and sexual dysfunction. Linn Goldberg, M.D., and Diane L. Elliot, M.D., codirectors of the Human Performance Laboratory at Oregon Health Sciences University, and coauthors of *The Healing Power of Exercise* (John Wiley, 2000), maintain that current research shows that 90 to 120 minutes a week of moderate exercise will make you feel better and will slow down your internal biological clock. This can delay and in some cases reverse the aging process. Dr. Goldberg and Dr. Elliot have found from their research that being actively involved in a regular program of physical exercise can:

- Increase the life span.
- Reduce the chance of developing heart disease.
- Reduce the risk of stroke.
- Lower the risk of developing certain cancers.
- Prevent and treat high blood pressure.
- Prevent and treat diabetes.
- Burn fat and build muscle.
- Strengthen the bones.
- Improve the cholesterol and triglyceride levels.
- Prevent and reduce back problems.
- Reduce stress, anxiety, and depression.
- Boost energy levels.

How does all this tie in with sexual fitness? According to sex therapist Roger Libby, Ph.D., "To fully enjoy our sexual potential and pleasure, we must vigorously increase our endeavors to maintain our overall health." Dr. Libby insists that sexual health is part of general wellness. In other words, living well may be our best defense against many of the problems associated with sexual dysfunction.

Elliott J. Howard, M.D., a cardiologist at Lenox Hill Hospital in New York City and the author of *Health Risks* (H.P. Books, 1987), compares exercise to the money in a bank account. Dr. Howard, who in 1970 established a foundation for the study of exercise, stress, and the heart, maintains that the benefits of exercise are not guaranteed forever. Unlike the money in a bank account that begins collecting interest immediately, exercising in the early years does not ensure fitness in the later years. Dr. Howard reminds us that we need to exercise regularly to reap any long-term benefits. He says, "Over a lifetime, a body that is exercised on a routine basis will remain in a young and healthy state for a longer period of time."

In this chapter, we will discuss exercise, sexercise, and their benefits.

## Maximum Sensory Enjoyment

Besides eating right, exercising may be the most important thing you can do to remain sexually vibrant throughout your lifetime. Research clearly shows a strong correlation between many of today's degenerative illnesses and diminished sexual response. Why are so many degenerative conditions linked with sexual disorders? Because many degenerative illnesses involve blood vessel constriction, which hampers proper blood flow to the genitals.

Dr. Jennifer Berman and Dr. Laura Berman maintain that exercise increases the blood flow to the pelvic area and genitals. These two researchers claim that there are two very important ways in which regular exercise contributes to sexual health. First, it causes the body to release endorphins, which helps you to relax, fosters a sense of well-being, and gets you in the mood to engage in sexual contact. Endorphins are powerful brain chemicals that make you feel good, act as natural painkillers, and promote feelings of excitement, euphoria, happiness, and exhilaration. Second, exercise—especially brisk aerobic exercise—helps increase the blood flow to all the parts of the body, including the pelvic area and the sexual organs. To truly enjoy a sexual experience, proper blood flow and good sensory nerve function are crucial.

The Drs. Berman call exercise, because of this natural flow of blood into the pelvic and genital area, a kind of "natural Viagra." It is this unimpeded flow of blood that contributes to the strength and firmness of male erections. It is also this uninterrupted blood flow to the female sexual organs that heightens the physical pleasure and sensual feelings caused by sexual contact. Both the male and female responses to sexual stimuli are clearly enhanced by proper blood flow and circulation.

## Exercise, Flexibility, and Energy

Besides causing the release of endorphins, exercise has two other important effects that will enhance your sexual pleasure. These two effects are improved flexibility and increased energy. According to Richard Smith, in *The Dieter's Guide to Weight Loss During Sex* (Workman Publishing, 1978), when we engage in sexual activity, we tend to transform our mental, emotional, and psychological desires into physical goals. In many cases our goal is to reach a higher level of physical adeptness. However, regardless of our shape, size, and physical condition, we push ourselves to accomplish unrealistic sexual feats at times. Smith says:

> It is during sex that our bodies do, or at least try to do, the most magical and wonderful things. Lack of preparation can lead to shortness of breath, failure to respond to your partner's strokes and an intense desire to do nothing but stare at television and all this after just four minutes of foreplay.

Let's face the facts: To experience the sensory reactions, sexual satisfaction, and gusto that we mentally visualize, we need energy. To become an exciting and fully functional sexual being, one of the most important things you can do for yourself is get your body moving.

## Exercise and Weight Loss

One of the greatest benefits of regular physical activity is a sleek, slender body. From a sexual standpoint, humans tend to look at the physical body before the mind. We are bombarded with messages each and every day that being physically attractive is related to being sexual. Being physically attractive doesn't mean you will have the psychological or emotional ability to sustain a lustful, happy sexual relationship with your partner. However, regular sexual intercourse can help you control your weight. Sexual intercourse is undoubtedly the most pleasurable exercise you can do. In their early studies, Masters and Johnson found that both men and women expend an appreciable amount of energy during sexual intercourse. In fact, these researchers found that, depending on the duration, position, and vigor of the sexual encounter, we can burn anywhere from 7 to 25 calories per hour.

So, besides keeping you healthy, regular sexual intercourse can help you maintain your physical attractiveness.

## Exercise and Mortality

One of the most exciting fields of study emerging today is that of anti-aging. It is a well-known fact that regular exercise not only helps us stay fit and maintain attractive slender bodies, but also helps us to live longer. While this fact may be yesterday's news, current research suggests that not only can sex help you cope better during periods of stress, elevate your mood, help you lose weight, and boost your overall feelings of well-being, it is also linked to decreased mortality, according to an article, "Sex and Death: Are They Related? Findings from the Caerphilly Cohort Study," published in the *British Medical Journal* in 1997. The authors of the study concluded that males who had at least two orgasms a week have decreased mortality (death) rates. Simply put, men who remain sexually active live longer. Michael Roizen, M.D., author of *Real Age: Are You as Young as You Can Be?* (HarperCollins, 1999), states that "the Caerphilly Study is the strongest proof we have that sex can actually help us get younger and stay younger." The Caerphilly study was conducted in the Welsh town of Caerphilly and five neighboring villages. The investigators found a definitive link between orgasmic frequency and overall life span in the 2,512 men studied.

Early studies such as the Duke University First Longitudinal Study of Aging, which was conducted in the 1950s and followed 270 men and women over a 25-year period, found that the frequency of sexual intercourse was a true predictor of an individual's longevity. Dr. Roizen says, "I believe so much in the therapeutic value of sex that I even prescribe sex for several of my patients, going so far as to write it out on a prescription pad!"

In addition, John Gittleman, associate professor of biology at the University of Virginia, says that "sexual activity appears to be a key factor in how the immune system develops." These findings, reported in the journal *Science* in November 2000, were obtained by comparing 20 years of data on the average white blood cell counts of 41 different primate species. The study suggests that the more active sexually you are, the more immune you are to disease.

## Exercise and Sexercise

Based on the benefits that regular exercise can contribute to your sexual health, you may want to focus your efforts on increasing the aerobic capacity of your lungs and heart, your flexibility, your stamina, and the blood flow to your genitals. The first three goals can be achieved through a number of different activities, such as:

- Aerobics
- Ballet
- Baseball
- Basketball
- Bowling
- Cycling
- Dancing
- Gardening
- Golfing
- Hiking
- Jogging
- Karate
- Racquetball
- Sexual intercourse
- Skating
- Skiing
- Swimming
- Tennis
- Walking
- Weight training

The most important thing to do is to keep moving. Take the stairs instead of the elevator, park your car at the far end of the mall, walk to work, use a push mower instead of a riding mower. Stuart M. Berger, M.D., the author of *Forever Young* (William Morrow, 1989), reminds us that it is regular exercise, not strenuous exercise, that is the key to health and longevity. Dr. Berger maintains that you actually get the greatest benefits when you change from no activity to moderate activity, rather than when you go from moderate activity to high activity.

But are there exercises that can be done that will specifically increase the blood flow to the sexual organs? And since the sex organs are composed of muscle tissue, are there exercises that will strengthen and increase the flexibility of the sexual apparatus?

The answer to both these questions is yes! Scientifically known as sexercises, a number of routines have proven to be very effective at restoring sexual potency and vitality to the sexual organs. While we do not have the room to cover all of the routines recommended by sex therapists today, we will discuss one of the most popular and widely used—Kegel exercises.

## Kegel Exercises

Kegel exercises are named after gynecologist Arnold Kegel, M.D. Dr. Kegel discovered in the 1950s that when the pubococcygeous muscle, commonly referred to as the PC or pelvic floor muscle, is exercised daily, pregnant women can control their bladders better. Kegel exercises also are recommended to men with incontinence problems due to prostate disorders. Urologists have found that Kegel exercises massage the prostate gland. This helps the body eliminate stagnant prostatic fluid.

How do Kegel exercises increase sexual gratification? The PC muscle, which helps expel urine from the bladder, is also the muscle that is responsible for the power and explosive nature of ejaculation in men and the intensity of orgasms in women.

Imagine the tension and power you feel when you pull back the string of a bow to fire an arrow. Visualize the force, power, and speed with which the arrow leaves the bow and hits the intended target. This can be compared to the moment right before you ejaculate or have an orgasm. Is your stream or flow continuously strong, robust, and full of power and excitement? Or after reaching this climactic stage, are you left wondering what all the hoopla is about?

By keeping the PC muscles in shape, you can enjoy the explosive orgasms that nature intended. To find your PC muscle, the next time you urinate, start and stop the flow of your urine. The muscle you are clinching to do this is your PC muscle. Dr. Ruth Westheimer claims that when women learn how to use this muscle, they can enhance both their own pleasure during sexual intercourse and their partner's. She says that stimulation of the PC muscle can create a sense of exhilaration and intense pleasure in a woman. Using the tightening and relaxing action of Kegel exercises during intercourse when the erect penis is inside the vagina, a woman can boost the sensations both she and her partner experience.

Kegel exercises can be done almost anywhere and anytime: at work, at home, while driving, while talking with a friend, while watching television, while taking a bath. To do them, clinch and relax your PC muscle about ten times in a row. Hold each clinch for 3 to 5 seconds. Do this at least five times a day. Work gradually up to clinching your PC muscle at least thirty times in a row, holding each clinch for 3 to 5 seconds, three times a day.

Dr. Laura E. Corio suggests doing at least ten repetitions twice a day in the beginning, holding each clinch for 2 or 3 seconds. She recommends working up to as many as possible, shooting for fifty daily. According to Dr. Corio, you will notice a difference in a few weeks.

Kenneth Goldberg, M.D., medical director of the Male Health Institute at Baylor Health Center at Irving-Coppell, Texas, has found that men generally see improvement in 4 to 6 weeks.

You should now have a clearer picture of why and how a solid regime of physical exercise can help you maintain an active, enjoyable life, as well as a rewarding sex life. It should also be evident that without some sort of exercise routine, the big four—aerobic capacity, blood flow, energy, and flexibility—are going to be problems. Exercise will increase your chances of maintaining a healthy sexual appetite throughout your lifetime.

In the next chapter, we will take a look at another important aspect of sexual health—stress and how well you adapt to it. We will examine stress and stressors and how they can literally kill your sex drive.

# 15

# Sometimes You Just Have to Unplug

*Those whose emotional lives are stuck on anger, frustration, fear, resentment, or other negative attitudes live in a continuous mode of physiological defense, whether they are aware or not. They are under unrelenting internal stress. They don't relax even when they're asleep. During sleep, physiology is run exclusively by the subconscious mind; the body is on automatic pilot. This stress physiology dramatically influences how the body functions.*

M. Ted Morter Jr., M.D.
*Your Health, Your Choice* (Lifetime Books, 1993)

On *Oprah* in March 2001, Phillip McGraw, Ph.D., author of *Strategies: Doing What Works, Doing What Matters* (Hyperion, 1999), told a couple experiencing a sexual setback "Only you can disconnect!" Take a moment and think about this powerful statement. Compare it to the quote from Dr. M. Ted Morter at the top of this page. Then ask yourself the following questions:

1. Which statement applies to me?
2. Does my sex life revolve around my work or my children's schedule?
3. Am I generally too tired or stressed to think about sex?
4. Do I avoid setting aside or planning time to be alone with my partner?

5. Am I opposed to suggestions from my partner about enhancing our sex life?
6. Have I stopped initiating sexual contact?
7. Has there been a decline in my sex drive over the last several months?
8. Are my sexual encounters with my partner dull and unfullfilling?
9. Am I experiencing bouts of anxiety, depression, insomnia, and increased weight gain?
10. Are emotional setbacks and arguments affecting my ability and/or desire to perform sexually?
11. Am I experiencing food cravings, light-headedness, and problems with concentration?
12. Am I having muscle and joint pain and suffering from unexplained bouts of generalized fatigue?
13. Have my eating habits recently become erratic?
14. Is my participation in sex no longer an expression of my innermost feelings, but rather an expression of guilt or responsibility?
15. Do I forgo sexual pleasure because I am a workaholic?

If you answered yes to at least half of questions 2 through 15, you may be suffering from a sexual energy crisis. A sexual energy crisis is caused by what healthcare professionals refer to as stress overload. Stress overload results when your daily life events or circumstances become overwhelming.

Just what is stress and how does it affect your internal biological mechanisms? More important here, how can stress turn a robust sexual appetite completely off? Is it stress from within or from outside yourself that derails sexual desire? Answering the questions in this paragraph is the goal of this chapter. Additionally, we will look at the concept of "adaptation" and at how it correlates with diminished sexual capacity. We will also discuss how you can use stress to your advantage and reconnect to your sexual communication system.

## Stress—A Silent Killer

According to Paul A. Jones, M.D., chief fellow of cardiovascular medicine at Loyola University Medical Center in Chicago, stress is an imbalance between the emotional, psychological, and physical demands on an individual and the individual's ability to cope with them.

Consider the following list of disorders that have been linked to stress:

- Accelerated aging
- Adrenal exhaustion
- Arteriosclerosis
- Arthritis
- Asthma
- Cancer
- Chronic fatigue syndrome
- Depression
- Diabetes
- Digestive disorders
- Diminished libido
- Elevated cholesterol levels
- Fibromyalgia
- Heart disease
- High blood pressure
- Hormonal imbalances
- Impotency
- Immune system dysfunctions
- Infertility
- Insomnia
- Kidney damage
- Menstrual irregularities
- Migraine headaches
- Strokes
- Ulcers

Based on this short list, it would appear that as a species we have not learned how to cope with the physical or psychological effects of stress.

As we have already discussed, our sexual capabilities are among the last bodily functions that will decay. A body racked with heart disease, diabetes, high blood pressure, arthritis, AIDS, and even cancer can still maintain its sexual prowess up to a point. However, a body under attack from uncontrolled stress and anxiety will eventually throttle down and lose its energy capacity.

## The Many Faces of Stress

Many people relate stress with the nervous tension caused by an outside force such as an emotional confrontation or argument. It is this misconception that can cause you to overlook many of the different types of stressors that pervade your everyday life. Noise, illegal drugs, chronic pain, depression, prescription medication, insomnia, obsessive-compulsive behavior, alcohol abuse, loneliness, failure at work, lack of exercise, and poor nutritional choices are all types of stressors.

Most people are unaware of another very important characteristic of stress. According to Dr. Hans Selye, it is immaterial whether a stressor is pleasant or unpleasant. In his book *Stress Without Distress,* (Lippincott and Crowell, 1974) Selye claims that the only thing important about a stressor is the intensity of the demand it places on the body. He says that stress-producing factors, although different in nature and source, all cause the body to react in a similar physical fashion. According to Marilyn Gilbert, M.S., a stress management consultant in Tucson, Arizona, the stress reaction initiates an irreversible cascade of some 1,400 neurohormonal events at least 50 times a day.

The body usually finds a way to adapt, however. This is known as adaptive stress. Depending on the degree of the stress, the nervous and endocrine systems swing into high or low gear. Dr. Selye calls the body's reaction to stress the general adaptation system or the stress syndrome.

## The Body's Response to Stress

Researchers now know that it is the nervous system that "sounds the alarm" that a stressor has been encountered. In response to the alarm, the body's internal systems prepare to do battle with the stressor. Following are some of the negative reactions caused by what the body perceives to be a threat to its normal state of equilibrium:

- Endorphins are released.
- Heart rate increases.
- Digestion stops.
- Blood pressure rises.
- Blood sugar levels rise.
- Adrenal glands begin working overtime.
- Blood vessels in the brain and skeletal muscles constrict.
- Insulin levels rise.
- Cholesterol and fat levels rise.

These reactions compose what Selye refers to as the alarm phase. The problem is that many of the disorders listed on page 199 can be traced back to this alarm phase. Increases in blood pressure, heart rate, cortisol production, blood sugar levels, insulin levels, and cholesterol production, along with a decrease in immunity and a complete slowdown of the digestive system can spell disaster.

All of this frantic activity is modulated by signals from the autonomic nervous system. The autonomic nervous system is responsible for bodily functions such as heart rate, blood pressure, and digestion. While these changes help the body prepare to meet the perceived challenge, they also increase your chances of becoming ill. Imagine leaving your car parked with the motor running for a substantial amount of time. Eventually the car will run out of gas, overheat, or just shut down. Naturopathic doctors use a theoretical model called the Naturopathic Model of Disease. This model shows how a body in optimal health begins its descent toward illness due to chronic stress, irritation, and inflammation of body systems and tissues. The constant distress will eventually disrupt or stifle what naturopathic physicians refer to as the body's vital life force. This will set up the system to age faster, shut down its communication system, and finally self-destruct. To protect itself and prevent this from happening, the body again shifts gears. The body works extremely hard to maintain what it believes is a state of external balance and harmony—in essence, a state of perfect health. It is precisely this invisible intelligence that Dr. Deepak Chopra and Dr. Norman Walker say exists within and outside of us. It is this vital force that is compromised and challenged by chronic stress.

## Stress, Resistance, and Adaptation

Biological researchers Paul M. Insel and Walton T. Roth, editors of *Core Concepts in Health* (Mayfield Publishing, 2001), define stress as the sum of the biological reactions to any stimulus—pleasant or unpleasant; physical, mental, or emotional; external or internal—that disturbs the organism's homeostasis. Homeostasis is a concept that was first proposed by nineteenth-century French physiologist Claude Bernard. Bernard believed that the most important shared feature of all living species was the need and ability to stabilize their internal environment under extenuating circumstances. In 1911, physiologist Walter B. Cannon of Harvard University first called this inborn mechanism "homeostasis."

In the second phase of the stress response, the body uses its energy and intelligence to regain homeostasis. It shifts gears and begins to make adjustments to adapt to the negative changes of the alarm stage. Dr. Selye referred to this phase as the "resistance phase" of stress.

The final phase of the stress response and another feature shared by all living matter is that of adaptation. Dr. Selye, in *Stress Without Distress,* insists that adaptation is what makes life possible. He says that the ability we have to adapt to changing conditions is actually the basis of homeostasis and of our resistance to stress. According to Dr. Morter, the body essentially operates in a minute-by-minute survival mode rather than a long-term survival mode. This is nature at its best.

Adaptation is a key reason we are able to remain energetic, sexually vibrant, and mentally focused even during times of stress. During the alarm stage, when our body is under constant stress, our energy demands increase to fuel and sustain us. Without fuel, we would experience a state of total exhaustion. How well your body is able to adapt to stressful challenges correlates to how well it can maintain its stress energy reserves. This is why learning how to manage your stress is so important to your general health as well as your sexual health.

## Stress and Sexuality

In addition to all the negative effects on individuals suffering from stress overload that we have already mentioned in this chapter, there also is a precipitous drop in the amount of sex hormones produced. Furthermore, evidence indicates that during periods of physical and emotional stress, including sex, unexplained bouts of amnesia can occur. This phenomenon is known as transient global amnesia. Researchers reported in the August 15, 1997 issue of the *Journal of Neurology, Neurosurgery, and Psychiatry* that these bouts of amnesia during sexual intercourse usually last from 30 to 60 minutes. Although the patients cannot remember the sexual encounter, they show no other signs of changes in consciousness or apparent neurological damage.

Leon Zussman, M.D., the former director of the Human Sexuality Center at the Long Island Jewish–Hillside Medical Center, found that stress can cause chemical changes that can profoundly affect sexual desire. Dr. Zussman conducted research on young men preparing to go to the front lines of combat during the Vietnam war. He found a marked increase in the soldiers' adrenaline levels that ultimately led to reduced testosterone levels. These young men had a significant drop in sexual interest. Dr. Zussman reported that after returning from battle, the men's body chemistry returned to normal and their sexual interest returned.

As you can see, stress can have dramatic negative affects on your body systems and vital organs. Energy, stamina, and a feeling of well-being promote sexuality and the need for human contact. According to Helen Singer Kaplan, M.D., Ph.D., director of the Sex Therapy and Education Program of the Payne Whitney Clinic of New York Hospital, depression, stress, and fatigue can have a devastating affect on sexual health.

Peter G. Hanson, M.D., author of *The Joy of Stress* (Andrews, McMeel and Parker, 1985), focuses on the subtle changes stress can cause in sexual behavior. He suggests that over time many couples do not notice the changes in their sexual habits, appetite, and frequency of sexual contact partly because of what he describes as a stress transformation. Your thoughts, your lifestyle, your personality, and your sexual habits all change gradually as part of your adaptation to the stress in your life.

## You Are What You Are Stressed About

Healthcare professionals believe that the longer you identify with the stress factors in your life, the more you become them. For example, some individuals cannot separate themselves from the disease or chronic condition they may have. Consequently, they use every moment and every ounce of energy to fix or deal with their physical or emotional trauma.

Researchers such as Deepak Chopra, Bernie Siegel, Joan Borysenko, Steven Locke, and Carl Simonton maintain that a stressful situation can become part of every structure, cell, neurotransmitter, and organ in our body. Dr. Siegel says that we store our life's events and experiences deep within the cellular recesses of our body. He adds that this should inspire us to start cleaning house to remove our painful old memories, which can damage our residence (our body) and thus destroy our sexual health. This new and exciting field that explores how the mind affects the physical body is called psychoneuroimmunology.

Holly Atkinson, M.D., a former medical reporter for the CBS Morning News, says that the first step in reducing one's stress load is to recognize it. Dr. Hanson claims that only by being aware of your stressors can you cope with them.

One way to take a look at the stressors in your life and their possible impact on your health is via the Holmes-Rahe Scale (see Appendix D).

Devised back in the 1960s by Dr. Thomas H. Holmes and colleagues at the University of Washington School of Medicine, this scale lists many of the common life events we experience. A numerical value is assigned to each event, representing the degree of stress the event usually causes in relation to the other events in the scale. Researchers have been able to show that individuals with a score of 300 or more have a 90 percent chance of developing some type of illness, possibly serious, within two years. Richard Earle, Ph.D., cofounder and director of the Canadian Institute of Stress, says that individuals with a score of 150 have a 33 percent chance of developing an illness. Dr. Earle adds that the Holmes-Rahe Scale has its limitation, since it rates the stressor rather than your reaction to it.

## Moving Toward Your Perception

Many health professionals who study mind-body medicine claim that we create our reality. While the Holmes-Rahe Scale has its merits, it doesn't measure how devastating or painful a particular life event may be. According to Insel and Roth in *Core Concepts in Health* some 2000 years ago the Roman emperor Marcus Aurelius said:

> If you are distressed by anything external, the pain is not due to the thing itself but to your estimate of it. This you have the power to revoke at any time.

This brings us full circle to Dr. Phillip McGraw's statement at the beginning of this chapter, but now expanded: Only you can disconnect from your sexual self and only you can reconnect with it!

Dharma Singh Khalsa, M.D., suggests in his book *Brain Longevity* (Warner Books, 1999) that our beliefs about stress are incorrect. Dr. Khalsa has found in his research that many individuals define stress as being caused by a force outside of ourselves and as causing us to feel distraught. Stress, unfortunately, is unavoidable. However, it can be good up to a certain point. It gets us moving, pushes us to meet our challenges mentally and physically. In connection with sex, the stress of not being able to perform well or of being rejected keeps us on our toes. It makes us buy flowers, plan romantic getaways, dress sexily, keep our bodies in shape, and adorn ourselves with soft silky scents.

Stress keeps us focused on living, participating, doing, and remaining sexually fit. This is the type of stress that Dr. Hanson wants us to embrace and to use to our advantage. It is your perception of a situation or event that makes it stressful. Learning to adapt your reaction to a particular stressor is the key to regaining your energy, your sexual vitality, and your sexual health.

## The Stressful Psychosexual Stages of Development

Sigmund Freud's theory concerning the psychosexual stages of development assumes that the early years of childhood play a critical role in human development. Freud was primarily concerned with personality development, the pathological outcomes of the failure to deal with conflict, and the problems associated with fixation (the tendency to stay at a particular stage of development), which can surface in adulthood. Contrary to Freud, psychologist Erik Erikson, Ph.D., author of *The Life Cycle Completed* (W.W. Norton, 1982), views personality as continuing its development throughout the life cycle. Erikson's view is much more optimistic. He believes that as individuals develop over the life cycle, they move toward healthy and positive resolutions of their identity and other life crises.

Robert A. Levine, Ph.D., author of *Culture, Behavior and Personality* (Aldine Publishers, 1979), examines the adaptive processes that we go through to become stabilized as we move from one stage of development to another. Stress in the alarm phase leaves us in a fixation stage. Instead of living outside of the stress, we live within it. We become it and eventually are consumed by it. This drains us of our passion for life, love, and human sexual contact. It causes us to disconnect.

Stress may be one of the most dangerous adversaries your sexual health will encounter. It has the ability to cause infertility, as well as amenorrhea (the sudden cessation of a woman's period). It can cause changes deep within your cells, in your DNA, and in your hormonal systems, literally zapping your energy and vital life forces.

Dr. Domeena Renshaw reminds us that sexual enjoyment requires time and relaxation. Dr. Howard Peiper and Nina Anderson say that "at the heart of sex is an odd, almost Zen-like irony." They claim that to perform well sexually, we must not try too hard. These authors insist that we have to relax, get out of our own way, and just let our sexual appetite and communication system do their job. What an impossible task this becomes when the body is under seige, overwhelmed by stress, tension, and fatigue. Susan Lark, M.D., author of *The Menopause Self-Help Book* (Celestial Arts, 1993), says that the energy that accumulates in the body to meet a perceived emergency has to be discharged in some way to bring the body back into balance. For 200 ways to naturally reduce your stress level, see Appendix E. And remember, depending on the severity of the stressful situation, there is one other way to reduce your stress level: have some sex. What a way to make stress your ally!

One of the most important things you can do to preserve your sexual health is to take control of the stress in your life instead of letting it control you. Envision the sexual relationship you want and deserve. Then take the necessary steps to remove the obstacles standing in your way.

# Conclusion

Roger J. Williams, Ph.D., author of *The Wonderful World Within You* (Bantam Books, 1977), says:

> In order to take care of one's complex physical equipment, it is necessary, at least partially, to understand it. If one is not willing to learn he or she must take the consequences. These may include living a life less rich in energy and statisfaction than it might have been.

Dr. Williams claims that developing and maintaining a healthy constitution is a life-long endeavor. He says that "there is no stage in life at which we can safely neglect the problem of proper maintenance."

When you regard sexuality from this viewpoint, the purely physical use of one's sexual apparatus seems limited. It becomes apparent that we must focus on our whole being to connect our physical and mental sexual capabilities. In fact, disregarding our being as a whole primes us for failure.

Study after study shows that Viagra and other drugs that just stimulate certain biological actions or reactions do not support the normal physiological mechanisms. Rather, they override the normal bodily processes, and thus become risky and dangerous to normal health and well-being. In the end, you not only compromise your sexual health, but your life.

Sex is more than the physical act. However, the physical act is extremely important. No matter your physical condition, political beliefs, social standing, economic status, or gender, your sexual performance is no doubt a concern. Like athletes, dancers, surgeons, astronauts, and singers, you wish to perform at a high level. Without a sexual-health plan in place, your sexual performance will give out slowly and silently. Should you focus on taking pills or injections to restore life to your clogged penile arteries? Should you take antidepressants to bring back those energy-filled orgasms and soulful sensory feelings? It should now be apparent to you why nonconventional and even many conventional healthcare professionals today believe that the complete medicalization of sexual dysfunction is inappropriate. It is important to look beyond the dysfunction, since, as stated by Dr. Williams, "to take care of one's complex physical equipment, it is necessary, at least partially, to understand it."

In the absence of any biological defects, you are capable of having and enjoying a vibrant sex life your whole life. Start becoming aware of the changes that occur during the different life stages. Begin incorporating some of the therapies discussed in this book. You are the one who will actually determine whether or not your sexual capabilities will remain at peak efficiency. You, more than the biological changes that you will experience, will make the difference in your enjoyment of your sexual capabilities in a peak fashion for life!

# THE HOLISTIC SEXUAL
# HEALTH DIRECTORY

# Organizations

American Academy of Anti-Aging
  Medicine
401 North Michigan Avenue
Chicago, IL 60611-6610
773-528-4333

The American Association of
  Naturopathic Physicians
2366 East Lake Avenue
Suite 204
Seattle, WA 98102
206-328-8310

American Foundation for
  Urologic Disease
300 West Pratt Street
Suite 401
Baltimore, MD 21201
410-468-1800

Association of Holistic Healing
  Centers
109 Holly Crescent
Suite 201
Virginia Beach, VA 23451
844-422-9022

Complementary and Alternative
  Medicine at the NIH
Office of Alternative Medicine
  Clearing House
P.O. Box 8218
Silver Spring, MD 20907-8218
888-644-6226

Menstrual Health Foundation
104 Petaluma Avenue
Sebastopol, CA 95472
707-829-2744

Office of Alternative Medicine
900 Rockville Pike
Building 51, Room 5B-37
Mailstop 2182
Bethesda, MD 29829
888-644-6226

Sexuality Information and
  Education Council of the
  United States
130 West 42nd Street
Suite 350
New York, NY 10036-7802
212-819-9770

The American Association of Sex
Educators, Counselors and
Therapists/ Society for the
Scientific Study of Sex
P.O. Box 238
Mount Vernon, IA 52314-0238
319-895-8407

The Sexual Health Network
3 Mayflower Lane
Huntington, CT 06484
203-924-4623

# For Men

Impotence Foundation
P.O. Box 60260
Santa Barbara, CA 93160
800-221-5517

Impotence Institute of America
8201 Corporate Drive
Suite 320
Landover, MD 20785-2229
800-699-1603

Men Center Counseling
1600 D Beekman Place, N.W.
Washington, DC 20009
202-393-3300

Men's Health Network
310 D Street, N.E.
Washington, DC 20002
202-543-6461

The Men's Center Foundation
2931 Shattuck Avenue
Room 102
Berkeley, CA 94705
510-644-0107

The Northern California Men's
Center
621 East Campbell Avenue
Suite #14
Campbell, CA 95008
408-379-4212

# For Women

American Medical Women's
  Association
801 North Fairfax
Suite 400
Alexandria, VA 22314
703-549-3864

American Menopause
  Foundation, Inc.
The Empire State Building
350 Fifth Avenue
Suite 2822
New York, NY 10118
212-714-2398

Asian Health Project
T.H.E. Clinic for Women Inc.
3860 West Martin Luther King
  Boulevard
Los Angeles, CA 90008
213-295-6571

Her Place: Health Enhancement
  and Renewal for Women Inc.
2700 Tibbets Drive
Suite 100
Bedford, TX 76022
817-355-8008

National Women's Health
  Network
514 10 Street, N.W.
Suite 400
Washington, DC 20004
202-347-1140

Women's Health America
P.O. Box 9690
Madison, WI 53715
608-833-9102

# Treatment Centers

The Atkins Center for
  Complementary Medicine
152 East 55th Street
New York, NY 10022
212-758-2110

The Gerber Medical Clinic
3670 Grant Drive
Reno, NV 89509
775-826-1900


Health Connections Center
530 South 2nd Street
Philadelphia, PA 19147
215-627-6000
http://www.members:aol.com/heal
  thcctr
Specializes in colon therapy.


The Integrative Medicine Clinic
The University of Arizona College
  of Medicine
P.O. Box 245153
Tucson, AZ 85724-5153
520-694-6555

King County Natural Medicine
  Clinic
(In Association with Bastyr
  University and Community
  Health Centers of King County)
8309 South 259th Street
Kent, WA 98031
253-852-2866


The Kinsey Institute Clinic
Indiana University Health Center,
  4th Floor
600 North Jordan Street
Bloomington, IN 47405
812-855-3878


The Male Health Center
Kenneth A. Goldberg, M.D.
5744 LBJ Freeway
Suite 100
Dallas, TX 75240
972-490-MALE

Male Sexual Dysfunction Clinic
3401 North Central Avenue
Chicago, IL 60634
800-788-CURE

National Health East
National College of Naturopathic
    Medicine
4231 SE Market Street
Portland, OR 97216

Our Lady of Lourdes Wellness
    Center
900 Haddon Avenue
Suite 100
Collingswood, NJ 08108
856-869-3125
http://lourdeswellnesscenter.org

Parcells Cleanse Center
P.O. Box 2129
Santa Fe, NM 87504
800-871-6784

The Sixth Patriarch Zen Center
2584 Martin Luther King Way
Berkeley, CA 94704-4704
504-486-1762
Does personal energy analysis.

# Hot Lines

Impotence Hotline
800-221-5517

Impotence Information Center
800-843-4315

Men's Hotline
888-636-2636

Prostate Information Hotline
800-543-9632

Natural Library of Medicine
301-496-6308

Physicians for Alternative
  Medicine
800-717-5649

World Research Foundation
818-999-5483
Note: Will mail out packets of information on nonconventional treatment options for specified conditions.

Male Sexual Dysfunction Clinic
  of Chicago
800-788-CURE (2873)

Athena Institute for Women's
  Wellness
610-827-2200
Provides information on pheromones.

Menopause
800-222-4767

Sex Therapist Hotline
800-843-7274
Note: A referral counselor will speak personally with you at no charge to help you find the most appropriate sex therapist or resource in your area.

The M.D.'s Holistic Health Line:
  900-GET-WELL

# Sources for Sexual Enhancement Appliances and Erotica

Adam and Eve
P.O. Box 800
Carrboro, NC 27510
800-274-0330

Betty Dodson Workshop
P.O. Box 9933
Murray Hill Station
New York, NY 10156
888-558-9778
866-877-9676

Eve's Garden
119 West 57th Street #420
New York, NY 10019
810-848-3837

Frederick's of Hollywood
P.O. Box 229
Hollywood, CA 90078-0229
800-323-9525

Intimate Treasures
P.O. Box 77902
San Francisco, CA 94107
415-863-5002

Leisure Time Products
P.O. Box M827
Gary, IN 46401-9900
800-874-8960

Romantic Fantasy
Donnelly Enterprises
8320 Denise Drive
Seminole, FL 33777
727-393-9646

Sexuality Boutique
318 Harvard Street
Suite 32
Brookline, MA 02446
617-731-2626

# Suggested Reading

Adams, R., *Miracle Medicine Foods,* West Nyack, NY: Parker Publishing, 1977.

Airola, P., *Juice Fasting,* Phoenix, AZ: Health Plus Publishers, 1971.

Airola, P., *Sex and Nutrition,* Phoenix, AZ: Health Plus Publishers, 1970.

Bechtrel, S., Stains, L. R., and the editors of Men's Health Books, *Sex: A Man's Guide,* New York: The Berkley Publishing Group, 1996.

Beling, S., *Power Foods,* New York: HarperCollins, 1997.

Bender, S. D., *The Power of Perimenopause: A Women's Guide to Physical and Emotional Health During the Transitional Decade,* New York: Three Rivers Press, 1998.

Berman, J., and Berman, L., *For Women Only,* New York: Henry Holt, 2001.

Bernie, Z., *The New Male Sexuality,* New York: Bantam Doubleday Dell, 1993.

Bieler, H. G., *Food Is Your Best Medicine,* New York: Random House, 1965.

Bieler, H. G., and Nichols, S., *Dr. Bieler's Natural Way to Sexual Health,* Los Angeles, CA: Charles Publishing, 1972.

Boston Women's Health Collective: *Our Bodies, Ourselves for the New Century*, New York: Simon & Schuster, 1993.

Brauer, A. P., *Extended Sexual Orgasm*, New York: Warner Books, 2000.

Cheung, T., *Androgen Disorders in Women*, Alameda, CA: Hunter House, 1999.

Chia, M., and Abrams, D., *The Multi-Orgasmic Man*, San Francisco: HarperCollins, 1997.

Chopra, D., *Ageless Body, Timeless Mind*, New York: Harmony Books, 1993.

Corio, L. E., *The Change Before the Change*, New York: Bantam Books, 2000.

Corn, L., *The Great American Sex Diet*, New York: William Morrow, 2001.

Cranton, E., *Bypassing Bypass*, Trout Dale, VA: Medex Publishers, 1997.

Crenshaw, T. L., *The Alchemy of Love and Lust*, New York: G. P. Putnam's Sons, 1996.

Diamond, J., *Male Menopause*, Naperville, IL: Source Books, 1997.

Dodson, B., *Sex for One*, New York: Harmony Books, 1987.

Dudley, D., *Super Potency*, New York: Warner Books, 1992.

Fry, K., and Wingo, C., *Menopause Naturally*, Green Bay, WI: Impakt Publications, 2000.

Garrison, O., *Tantra: The Yoga of Sex*, New York: Harmony Books, 1983.

Gittleman, A. L., *Super Nutrition for Men*, Garden City Park, NY: Avery, 1999.

Gittleman, A. L., *Super Nutrition for Men and the Women Who Love Them*, New York: M. Evans and Co., 1996.

Gittleman, A. L., *Super Nutrition for Menopause*, Garden City Park, NY: Avery, 1996.

Godek, G., *1001 Ways to Be Romantic*, Naperville, IL: Casa Blanca Press, 2000.

Gould, S. J., *Time's Arrow, Time's Cycle,* Boston: Harvard University Press, 1987.

Graber, G. K., and Gerber, B., *Women's Orgasm,* New York: Warner Books, 1975.

Haas, E. M., *Detox Diet: A How-To Guide for Cleansing the Body of Toxic Substances,* Berkeley, CA: Celestial Arts, 1997.

Hausman, P., and Hurley, J. B., *The Healing Foods,* Emmaus, PA: Rodale Press, 1989.

Hewitt, J., *Natural Foods Cookbook,* New York: Avon Books, 1971.

Hooper, A., *Great Sex Games,* New York: Dorling Kindersley, 2000.

Hunter, B T., *The Natural Foods Cookbook,* New York: Pyramus Books, 1961.

Keesling, B., *Sexual Pleasure,* Alameda, CA: Hunter House, 1993.

Keller, L., *Report 2000: A Man's Guide to Women,* Emmaus, PA: Rodale Press, 1999.

Kline, G., and Graber, B., *Woman's Orgasm,* New York: Warner Books, 1975.

Kulvinskas, V., *The Lovers Diet,* Hot Springs, AR: Ihopea, 1998.

Lee, W. H., and Lee, L., *The Book of Practical Aromatherapy,* New Canaan, CT: Keats Publishing, 1994.

Lee, W. H., and Lee, L., *Herbal Love Potions,* New Canaan, CT: Keats Publishing, 1991.

Lloyd, J. E., *52 Saturday Nights,* New York: Warner Books, 2000.

Masters, W., and Johnson, V., *Human Sexual Inadequacy,* Boston: Little, Brown, 1970.

McGraw, P.C., *Strategies: Doing What Works, Doing What Matters,* New York: Hyperion, 1999.

Mobley, D. F., and Wilson, S. K., *Reversing Impotence Forever!* Alvin, TX: Swan Publishing, 1995.

Morgan, B., and Morgan, R., *Brainfood,* Tucson, AZ: The Body Press, 1987.

Morin, J., *The Erotic Mind: Unlocking the Inner Sources of Sexual Passion and Fulfillment,* New York: HarperCollins, 1995.

Peiper, H., and Anderson, N., *Natural Solutions for Sexual Dysfunction,* East Canaan, CT: Safe Goods, 1998.

Penny, A., *How to Make Love to a Man,* New York: Dell Books, 1987.

Pierrako, S. E., and Saly, J., *Creating Union: The Pathwork of Relationship,* Del Mar, CA: Pathwork Press, 1993.

Quillman, S., *Every Woman's Guide to Sexual Fulfillment,* New York: Simon & Schuster, 1997.

Redmon, G. L., *Energy for Life,* Bloomingdale, IL: Vital Health, 2000.

Redmon, G. L., *Managing and Preventing Prostate Disorder,* Prescott, AZ: Hohm Press, 2000.

Riley, M., Kahn, R., and Foner, A. (eds.) *Age and Structural Lag,* New York: John Wiley, 1994.

St. Claire, O., *Unleashing the Sex Goddess in Every Woman,* New York: Harmony Books, 1996.

Saraswati, S., and Avinasha, B., *Jewel in the Lotus: The Tantric Path to Higher Consciousness,* Taos, NM: Sunstar, 1996.

Silver, H., *The Body-Smart System: The Complete Guid to Cleansing and Rejuvenation,* New York: Bantam Books, 1990.

Simopoulos, A P., Herbert, V., and Jacobson, B., *Genetic Nutrition: Designing a Diet Based on Your Family Medical History,* New York: Macmillan, 1993.

Starr, B. D., and Weiner, M. B., *Sex and Sexuality in the Mature Years,* New York: Stein and Day, 1981.

Taormino, T., *The Ultimate Guide to Anal Sex for Women,* San Francisco: Cleis Press, 1998.

Townsley, C., *Cleansing Made Simple,* Littleton, CO: LFH Publishing, 1997.

Wade, C., *Health Secrets from the Orient,* West Nyack, NY: Parker Publishing, 1973.

Wade, C., *Inner Cleansing,* Paramus, NJ: Prentice-Hall, 1992.

Walker, M., *The Chelation Way: The Complete Book of Chelation Therapy,* Garden City Park, NY: Avery, 1990.

Walker, M., *Sexual Nutrition,* Garden City Park, NY: Avery, 1993.

Walker, N. W., *Fresh Vegetable and Fruit Juices,* Norwalk, CT: Norwalk Press, 1970.

Warmbrand, M., *The Encyclopedia of Health and Nutrition,* New York: Pyramid Books, 1962.

Watson, C., *Love Potions,* Los Angeles, CA: Putnam Publishing, 1993.

Weil, A., *Eating Well for Optimum Health,* New York: Alfred A. Knopf, 2000.

Wright, J., and Morgenthaler, J., *Natural Hormone Replacement,* Petaluma, CA: Smart Publications, 1997.

Wuh, H.C.K., *Sexual Fitness,* New York: G. P. Putnam's Sons, 2001.

Wurtman, J., *Managing Your Mind and Mood Through Food,* New York: Rawson Associates, 1986.

Yeager, S. and the editors of Prevention Health Books, *The Doctor's Book of Food Remedies,* Emmaus, PA: Rodale Press, 1998.

Zolbrod, A. P., *Sex Smart: How Your Childhood Shaped Your Sexual Life and What to Do About It.* Oakland, CA: New Harbinger Publications, 1998.

Zonderman, J., and Shader, L., *Nutritional Diseases,* New York: Twenty-First Century Books, 1993.

# Websites

ABCNEWS.com: Understanding Midlife Changes in Men
http://abcnews.go.com/section/living/dailynews/chat-diamond000614.
html

Alternative Medicine Digest
http://www.alternativemedicine.com

Chelation Therapy—Gale Encyclopedia of Medicine
http://www.findarticles.com/ct-dls/g2601/0002/2601002951/plarticle.
jhtml

Cleansing Network
http://hometown.aol.com/cleansingj/

Clear Path to Wellness
http://www.clearpathtowellness.com/

Colon Cleansing—Wholistic Health Solutions
http://www.bibkit.com/experts.html

EDTA Chelation Therapy
http://www.arxc.com/doctors/chelate.html

Holistic Medicine
http://www.holisticmedicine.com

Male Health
http://www.malehealthcenter.com

Men's Web
http://www.vix.com/menmag/

NIH Office of Dietary Supplements
http://ods.od.nih.gov/links-consumer.html
http://dietary-supplements.info.nih.gov

North America Menopause Society
http://menopause.org

Office of Alternative Medicine
http://www.altmed.od.nih.gov/

Office of Inspector General—U.S. Department of Health and Human Services
http://www.sba.gov/ignet/internal/hhs.html

Q and A With a Holistic Doctor
http://www.tripod.com/health/

Sexual Health
http://www.sexualhealth.com

Sexuality Information and Education Council of the United Sates
http://www.siecus

Sex Therapist Directories
http://madasafish.com/~answers/therapists/therapists-index.html

The Female Reproductive System
http://www.stdservices.on.net/management/checklist/cl-male.html

The Male Reproductive System
http://www.stdservices.on.net.management/checklist/cl-male.html

The National Institute on Aging
http://www.nih.gov/nia

The National Library of Medicine's Medline
http://ww.igm.nim.nih.gov/

The Society for Human Sexuality
http://www.sexuality.org

# Laboratories and Clinics

Aeron Life Cycles Laboratories
1933 Davis Street
Suite 310
800-631-7900
Test levels of testosterone, progesterone, and estrogen via saliva test
  kits.

Life Enhancement
P.O. Box 751390
Petaluma, CA 94975-9846
800-543-3873 or 707-762-6144
Offers variety of supplements designed to enhance the body's natural
  biochemical mechanisms, ranging from libido stimulation to anti-
  aging.

Medical Direct Corporation
22722 Vistawood Way
Boca Raton, FL 33428
800-658-2227
Offers Vitamed. Send in urine samples and a complete analysis of your
  specific nutrient levels is mailed back to you, usually within ten days.

Pantox Laboratories
4622 Santa Fe Street
San Diego, CA 92109
888-726-8698
Offers Pantox Antioxidant Profile (PAT), a test to determine how well
  the body's inborn antioxidant system is working.

Women's College Online Clinics and Programs
416-323-7731
**Note:** A program affiliated with Sunny Brook and Women's College
  Health Sciences Centre in Toronto, Canada, University of Toronto.
http://www.womenscollege.com/pages/clinics.html

Women's International Pharmacy
5708 Monona Drive
Madison, WI 53719-3152
800-279-5708

# Appendix A

# Foods for a Healthy Body

A well-nourished body is a key factor to maintaining your sexual health. There are literally hundreds of different foods that are touted for their ability to maintain and improve, and in some cases restore, libido and sex drive. For better sex, you may want to consider consuming generous helpings of the following:

| | | |
|---|---|---|
| Apples | Chocolate (sparingly) | Mussels |
| Asparagus | Dates | Oats |
| Beans | Essential fatty acids | Oranges |
| Bee pollen | Figs | Pumpkin seeds |
| Beets | Fish | Seaweed |
| Blueberries | Fresh fruits and veggies | Shellfish |
| Broccoli | Green tea | Tomatoes |
| Brown rice | Legumes | Wheat bran |
| Cacao beans | Melons | Whole-grain breads |
| Carrots | Molasses | Yogurt |

# Appendix B

# Foods for the Sexual Connoisseur

The following foods are not only good for your general health, but they are especially beneficial for your sexual health.

Bananas. Loaded with potassium; help regulate water balance. Believed to contain natural chelating agent that removes heavy metals from the arteries including the penile arteries.

Brewer's yeast, brazil nuts, tuna, bran, whole grains, sesame seeds. High in selenium, a mineral that helps modulate the immune function and that is the most abundant mineral found in the seminal fluid of men. When males ejaculate, levels of this mineral go down. It is vital to sexual functioning.

Chili peppers. Have a vasodilation effect on the sex gland arteries, the blood flow, and the circulation to the pelvic area, which facilitates hormone production.

Curries, pumpkin, squash, sunflower seeds. Rich in phosphorus, the first mineral found to be involved with mechanisms that control the sex drive.

Eggs, yellow fruits, acid vegetables. Rich in vitamin A, which helps to maintain testicular tissue.

Fish, cold water (salmon, mackerel, sardines). High in the omega-3 fatty acids, which reduce LDL levels, prevent atherosclerosis, assist proper cardiovascular function, and contribute to healthy skin.

Garlic and onions. Have natural immune-enhancing capabilities, act as natural antibiotics and chelating agents, and assist in the maintance of the pH balance.

Green leafy vegetables. Rich in antioxidants and bioflavonoids, which keep the arteries and veins elastic, provide flexibility to the joints by promoting collagen production, and keep the skin soft and wrinkle-free.

Green peppers, rose hips, strawberries, cantaloupe, broccoli. Rich in vitamin C, which assists sex-gland function. The sex glands will rob other body tissues of this nutrient if necessary.

Liver, brewer's yeast. Support adrenal gland function due to their high content of vitamin B, especially pantothenic acid. The B vitamins influence testosterone production.

Nuts and seeds. High in arginine, necessary for proper erections.

Oysters. Rich in zinc, vital to sexual maturation and strong sex glands. Zinc is abundant in the prostate gland.

Sarsaparilla. Contains cortin, which assists in modulating energy. Sarsaparilla also contains natural testosterone and progesterone.

Strawberries, apples. Contain elasic acids, which neutralize cancer-causing agents in tobacco smoke and processed foods.

Soy-based foods. Contain natural phytoestrogens, are low in fat, and may relieve or prevent menopausal symptoms.

Wheat germ. Rich in vitamin E, which helps alleviate hot flashes.

# Appendix C

# Liquid Sex Foods

If you need a sexual tune-up but are short on time, try the following drinks. They are safe, easy to prepare, inexpensive, and highly recommended.

**Green Thunder**
To an 8-ounce glass of water, add
1 teaspoon of mixed green foods and
1 teaspoon of honey
Stir vigorously. Drink two to three times daily.

**Instant Power Potion**
To an 8-ounce glass of fresh citrus juice, add
2 tablespoons of lecithin granules,
1 teaspoon of honey, and
½ teaspoon of brewer's yeast
Blend for 20 seconds. Drink slowly. This is a great rejuvenator that works almost instantly.

**The Energizer Bunny**
To an 8-ounce glass of carrot juice, add
1 teaspoon of liquid ginseng,
1 teaspoon of desiccated liver powder, and
2 teaspoons of blackstrap molasses
Stir. Drink twice daily.

**The Rotor Rooter**
To an 8-ounce glass of pineapple juice, add
2 teaspoons of apple cider vinegar,
2 teaspoons of vitamin C powder, and
2 teaspoons of lemon juice
Stir. Drink three times daily.

# Appendix D

# Holmes-Rahe Scale

The Holmes-Rahe Scale is an index of life events that affect most people's stress level. The life events are ranked according to how severely they generally affect the stress level. How well you adjust to these life events can have a direct bearing on the quality of your sexual health, as well as of your general health.

| LIFE EVENT | VALUE |
|---|---|
| Death of a spouse | 100 |
| Divorce | 73 |
| Marital separation | 65 |
| Jail term | 63 |
| Death of a close family member | 63 |
| Personal injury or illness | 53 |
| Marriage | 50 |
| Fired at work | 47 |
| Marital reconciliation | 45 |
| Retirement | 45 |
| Change in health of family member | 44 |
| Pregnancy | 40 |
| Sex difficulties | 39 |
| Gain of new family member | 39 |
| Business adjustment | 39 |
| Change in financial state | 38 |
| Death of a close friend | 37 |

| | |
|---|---|
| Change to different line of work | 36 |
| Change in number of arguments with spouse | 35 |
| Mortgage over one year's net salary | 31 |
| Foreclosure of mortgage or loan | 30 |
| Change in responsibilities at work | 29 |
| Son or daughter leaving home | 29 |
| Trouble with in-laws | 29 |
| Outstanding personal achievement | 28 |
| Spouse begins or stops work | 26 |
| Begin or end school | 26 |
| Change in living conditions | 25 |
| Revision of personal habits | 24 |
| Trouble with boss | 23 |
| Change in work hours or conditions | 20 |
| Change in residence | 20 |
| Change in schools | 20 |
| Change in recreation | 19 |
| Change in church activities | 19 |
| Change in social activities | 18 |
| Mortgage or loan less than one year's net salary | 17 |
| Change in sleeping habits | 16 |
| Change in number of family get-togethers | 15 |
| Change in eating habits | 15 |
| Vacation | 13 |
| Christmas | 12 |
| Minor violations of the law | 11 |
| Miscellaneous | |

Enter your total here.

If your total is over 300, then you have an 80 percent chance of a serious change in your health within the next year.

# Appendix E

# Two Hundred Ways to Naturally Reduce Your Stress Level

1. Take a walk.
2. Take a hot bath.
3. Call a friend.
4. Meditate.
5. Take a swim.
6. Run a few laps.
7. Have sex.
8. Listen to your favorite song.
9. Express yourself and your feelings.
10. Be honest with yourself.
11. Find a new hobby.
12. Get a massage.
13. Do some gardening.
14. Go to the beach.
15. Consider psychotherapy.
16. Consider biofeedback.
17. Learn yoga techniques.
18. Learn a new skill.
19. Develop friendships.
20. Teach a class.
21. Learn visualization techniques.
22. Dine out at your favorite restaurant.
23. Soak in your hot tub.
24. Relax in the sauna.
25. Take a steam bath.
26. Take a vacation.
27. Organize your life and daily schedule.
28. Learn how to accept others' shortcomings.
29. Go fishing.
30. Spend time with yourself.
31. Practice positive thinking.
32. Ask for help.
33. Break your routine.
34. Visit a friend.
35. Volunteer your time.
36. Read your favorite book.
37. Exercise, exercise, exercise.
38. Seek professional help.
39. Resolve past conflicts.
40. Make peace with yourself.
41. Seek spiritual guidance.
42. Modify and/or quit smoking.
43. Reduce your workload.
44. Go see a play.

45. Recognize your shortcomings.
46. Practice deep breathing exercises.
47. Hit a punching bag.
48. Do not overeat.
49. Listen to your favorite musical.
50. Forgive and forget.
51. Paint a picture.
52. Read works from your favorite poet.
53. Go see a movie.
54. Walk in the other person's shoes.
55. Don't take yourself too seriously.
56. Find humor in life's daily mishaps.
57. Become an effective listener.
58. Consider the attributes of St. John's wort for mild depression.
59. Consider the attributes of relaxation tapes.
60. Write down your concerns and make the necessary adjustments.
61. Diffuse a possible confrontation and talk it out.
62. Delegate when possible.
63. Manage your finances.
64. Reassess your life goals.
65. Join a support group.
66. Learn anger management techniques.
67. Live and let old grievances die.
68. Learn to forgive yourself for mistakes you've made.
69. Break problems into smaller parts then solve each part.
70. Go dancing.
71. Consider the attributes of reflexology.
72. Just say no, it's your time.
73. Take responsibility for your actions.
74. Establish regular sleeping patterns.
75. Reorganize your settings to reduce excess clutter.
76. Keep work problems at work.
77. Examine your beliefs and expectations.
78. Learn to ask for what you want sexually.
79. Discuss sexual concerns with your partner.
80. Remove the fear of rejection.
81. Remain focused on your goals.
82. Work on improving interpersonal and social skills.
83. Get plenty of rest.
84. Be flexible.
85. Learn how to accept constructive criticism.
86. Don't be afraid to succeed in reaching your goals.
87. Break a large complex task into smaller parts.
88. Be proud of what you have accomplished.
89. Identify your stressors.

90. Keep a journal listing the times of the day when you are most stressed.
91. Treat yourself to something.
92. Play a round of golf.
93. Join a health club.
94. Avoid alcohol, caffeine, and junk food.
95. Take 500 milligrams of vitamin C daily.
96. Consider taking a multivitamin.
97. Practice tai chi.
98. Make a career change if necessary.
99. Masturbate.
100. Turn off the television.
101. Do not take sleeping pills.
102. Know your biorhythmic cycles.
103. Take a scenic drive.
104. Define the right situation for you.
105. Use adaptogenic supplements to support adrenal functions.
106. Relax, relax, relax.
107. Utilize affirmations.
108. Consider color therapy.
109. Consider hydrotherapy.
110. Take a hot Epsom soak bath.
111. Don't procrastinate—do it now.
112. Seek crisis therapy in crisis-related situations.
113. Avoid environmental hazards.
114. Establish an emergency fund for unexpected expenditures.
115. Plan for success.
116. Lose those unwanted pounds.
117. Recognize your own attributes.
118. Let go—you cannot control every situation.
119. Know warning signs of stress overload.
120. Focus on overall health.
121. Avoid crash diets.
122. Measure success one day at a time.
123. Anticipate setbacks; focus on replanning.
124. Consider aromatherapy.
125. Go bowling.
126. Know your partner's sexual likes and dislikes.
127. Learn progressive muscular relaxation.
128. Consider self-hypnosis and autosuggestion.
129. Plan an intimate interlude.
130. Utilize stress reduction products such as indoor water fountains.
131. Reevaluate the perceived destruction of a crisis or life event.
132. Learn transcendental meditation.
133. Reduce your exposure to allergens.
134. Repeal the notion that your self-esteem is based on others' opinions of you.

135. Work hard to live; live to enjoy the fruit of your labor.
136. Consider using natural mood elevators such as tyrosine and 5-HTP.
137. Shoot some hoops with the guys or girls.
138. Schedule a racquetball session.
139. Stop, listen, and learn.
140. Stop to smell the roses.
141. Go to the ballet.
142. Seek professional help for sexual problems.
143. Become a big brother or a big sister.
144. Teach a class.
145. Write a letter to your spouse expressing your needs.
146. Plan a day of spontaneous activity with your lover.
147. Take the afternoon off and meet your partner or spouse before the kids get home.
148. Weather the emotional storm and move forward.
149. Try a little tenderness.
150. Say, "I am sorry. Please forgive me."
151. Nip personal conflicts in the bud.
152. Take a stand.
153. Live for today. Savor the possible tomorrows.
154. Be fruitful. Enjoy your sexuality.
155. Be considerate.
156. Dress to please.
157. Recognize your aggressive tendencies.
158. Make simple assertions instead of demanding ones.
159. Consider caring for a pet.
160. Resist the temptation to forestall pleasure due to other commitments.
161. Focus on your partner's strong points.
162. Compliment your partner when he or she has aroused your sexual interest.
163. Change your sexual environment.
164. Keep your doctor's appointment.
165. Say the words "I love you!"
166. Use the power of prayer.
167. Practice safe sex.
168. Pamper yourself.
169. Resist the notion that orgasm relates to sexual satisfaction.
170. Practice relaxing.
171. Learn mind-focusing techniques.
172. Know the warning signs of depression.
173. Establish daily detox routines.
174. Remember that past failures don't determine future success.
175. Create solutions.
176. Eat fresh wholesome foods.
177. Have regular prostate examinations.

178. Practice your sexercises.
179. Keep your elimination processes in good working order.
180. Have regular breast exams done.
181. Go to the spa.
182. Check in with your partner; remove doubt and uncertainty.
183. Trust your own judgment.
184. Hug your partner; hug your kids.
185. Explain why your point of view differs but respect others' rights to have opposing views.
186. Recognize and use voice volume-control techniques to diffuse stressful or hostile situations.
187. Be decisive. Speak clearly without long explanations.
188. Minimize negative gestures when communicating.
189. Make eye contact; be attentive to the discussion at hand.
190. Pace yourself; conserve energy.
191. Eat a nutritious breakfast.
192. Resist sugary snacks in between meals.
193. Eat at least three to four meals a day.
194. Take a daily multivitamin and mineral supplement.
195. Drink whole green food drinks in between meals.
196. Do not overeat; moderation is the key to health and vitality.
197. Avoid illicit drugs.
198. Use air filtration systems to minimize the effects of secondhand smoke.
199. Resist the notion that every minor detail must be accounted for.
200. Love thyself each and every day!

# Resource List

## Products for Women

Bio Femme IC™
Transdermal (PMS/Hot Flashes)
Saber Sciences Inc.
888-490-7300

Estroven
Amerifit
168 Highland Park Drive
Bloomfield, CT 06002
800-772-3472

Lady V
Smart Health
269 South Beverly Drive
Beverly Hills, CA 90212
201-236-9090

Natural Passion
Nature Plus
548 Broadhollow Road
Melville, NY 11747
www.naturesplus.com

Tigress
Action Labs
280 Adams Boulevard
Farmingdale, NY 11735
800-932-2593

Yohimbe for Women
Action Labs
280 Adams Boulevard
Farmingdale, NY 11735
800-932-2593

Biosis IC™
Transdermal Libido Crème
Saber Sciences Inc.
888-490-7300

Evalu 8™
Personal Home Hormone Profile
Life-Flo Health Care Products
P.O. Box 38099
Phoenix, AZ 85069
888-999-7440

Libido Formula (Women)
Transitions for Health Inc.
Portland, OR 97205
800-455-5182

Remifemin Plus
Enzymatic Therapy
825 Challenger Drive
Green Bay, WI 54311
920-469-1313

ViraMax for Women
Solaray Nutraceutical Corp.
Ogden, UT 84403
801-626-4956

## Products for Men

Andro Fuel, Tribulus Fuel and
Male Fuel
Twin Labs
150 Motor Parkway
Hauppauge, NY 11788
631-467-3146

Endo Screen™
Hormone Saliva Testing
Sabre Science Inc.
910 Hampshire Road
Suite P
Westlake Village, CA 91361
888-490-7300

Horny Goat Weed
Bodyonics LTD (Pinnacle)
140 Lauman Lane
Hicksville, NY 11801
516-822-1230

TestoSterol
Pyramid Nutrition
1200 Clint Moore Road #11
Boca Raton, FL 33487

800-491-1716
*www.pyramidnutrition.com*

Vigoril
ELS International
888-466-3622

Yohimbe (1500 and 2000)
Action Labs
280 Adams Boulevard
Farmingdale, NY 11735
800-932-2593

Cobra
Natural Balance
3155 North Commerce Court
Castle Rock, CO 80104
303-688-6633

Herbal V
Smart Health
269 South Beverly Drive
Beverly Hills, CA 90212
201-236-9090

Vero Max
Omni Nutraceuticals, Inc
P.O. Box 66457
Los Angeles, CA 90066
800-808-7266

Vira Max
Solaray Nutraceutical Corp.
Ogden, UT 84403
801-626-4956

## Products for Men and Women

All Natural Products, 516-741-3304
Aphrodisia Products, 800-221-9898
Aromatherapy International, 617-570-1792
Country Life Vitamins, 631-231-1031
Enzymatic Therapy, 920-469-1313 (enzymes, vitamins, accessory products)
Geni Soy Products, 888-GENISOY
Good and Natural Vitamins, 631-244-2041
Health From the Sun, 831-479-0227 (essential fatty acids)
Health Plus Inc., 909-627-9393 (fibers, cleansing products)
MD Labs, 800-255-2690 (detox teas)
Natures Plus, 631-293-0349 (herbs)
Naturopathic Research Inc., 941-426-3375 (mineral electrolytes)
Nature's Secret, 800-253-2673 (internal cleansing)
Nature's Way, 800-926-8883 (herbs)
New Chapter Inc., 800-543-7279 (vitamins, minerals, accessory products)
Now Foods, 630-545-9098 (vitamins, herbs, etc.)
Royal Brittany, 800-445-7137 (evening primrose oil)
Solgar Vitamin Co., 201-944-2311
Twin Labs Inc., 631-630-3490 (vitamins, hormones, accessories)

# Bibliography

Abbott, I., and Shimazu, C., "The Geographic Origin of the Plants Most Commonly Used for Medicine by Hawaiians," *Journal of Ethnopharmacology*, 1985: 14: 213–22.

Adamson, A., "Viagra Sales, Softening as HMO's and Women Beef: Perils Cited," *Philadelphia Daily News*, July 22, 1998, p. 2.

Airola, P., *Are You Confused?* Phoenix, AZ: Health Plus Publishers, 1980.

Airola, P., *How to Get Well*, Phoenix, AZ: Health Plus Publishers, 1989.

Airola, P., *Juice Fasting*, Phoenix, AZ: Health Plus Publishers, 1971.

Angelo, M., and Miller, A. L., "Nature's Pharmacy: Erectile Dysfunction," *Let's Live*, Los Angeles, CA, Vol. 69, No. 2, February 2001, p. 24.

Anthony, C. P., and Kolthoff, N. J., *Textbook of Anatomy and Physiology*, St. Louis, MO: C.V. Mosby Co., 1971.

Antoniak, M., "The Wisdom of Detoxification," *Vitamin Retailer*, East Brunswick, NJ, Vol. 4, No. 9, September 1997, pp. 26–28 (170).

Arnold, P., "Hormones: Anabolic and Catabolic An Overview," *Mind and Muscle Power*, New York, Vol. 1, No. 1, January 2000, pp. 74–76.

Atkins, H., *Women and Fatigue*, New York: Putnam, 1985.

Atkins, R. C., *Dr. Atkin's Vita-Nutrient Solution,* New York: Simon & Schuster, 1998.

Balch, P. A., and Balch, J. F., *Prescription for Nutritional Healing,* 3rd ed., New York: Avery, 2000.

Bardon, C. W., et al., "Androgens: Risk and Benefits," *Journal of Clinical Endocrinology and Metabolism,* 1991: 73 (1): 4–7.

Basson, R. J., Berman, A., Burnett, L., Derogatis, D., Ferguson, J., et al., "Report of the International Consensus Development Conference on Female Sexual Dysfunction: Definitions and Classifications." *Journal of Urology* 163 (2000): 889–93.

Basson, R. R., McInness, M.D., Smith, G., et al, "Efficacy and safety of sildenfil in estrogenized women with sexual dysfunction associated with female sexual arousal disorder," *Obstetrics and Gynecology* 95 (2000) 4 Supplement 1: S54.

Batchelder, H. J., "Velvet Antler: A Literature Review," *North American Elk Breeders Association,* Platte City, MO, 1999, website: www.naelk.org.

Belongie, L., "Natural Sexual Healing," *Health Supplement Retailer,* Phoenix, AZ, Vol. 7, No. 1, January 2001, pp. 52–54.

Bennett, M. L., "Vanity Medicine with Human Growth Hormone," *Nutrition Science News,* Boulder, CO, Vol. 5, No. 11, November 2000, pp. 456–60.

Berger, R. E., Berger, D., *Biopotency: A Guide to Sexual Success*, Emmaus, PA: Rodale Press, 1987.

Berger, S. M., *Forever Young,* New York: William Morrow, 1989.

Berger, S. M., *How to Be Your Own Nutritionist,* New York: William Morrow, 1987.

Berkow, R. (editor-in-chief), "Sexual Dysfunction in Women," *The Merck Manual of Diagnosis and Therapy* 15th ed., Rohway, NJ: Merck and Co., 1987, pp. 1653–60.

Berman, J., and Berman, L., *For Women Only,* New York: Henry Holt and Company, 2001.

Berman, J. R., Berman, L. A., Erbin, T. J., et al., "Female Sexual Dysfunction: Anatomy, Physiology, Evaluation, and Treatment Options," *Current Opinion Urology,* 1999 (9): 563–68.

Berry, L., *Internal Cleansing,* Roseville, CA: Prima Health, 2000.

Bieler, H. G., and Nichols, S., *Dr. Bieler's Natural Way to Sexual Health,* Los Angeles, CA: Charles Publishing Co., 1972.

Blum, D., *Sex on the Brain: The Biological Differences Between Men and Women,* New York: Penguin Publishing Group, 1997.

Blumfield, L. (ed), *The Big Book of Relaxation: Simple Techiniques to Control the Excess Stress in Your Life,* Roslyn, NY: The Relaxation Co. Inc., 1994.

Bortz, W. M., *Dare to Be 100,* New York: Simon & Schuster, 1996.

Bowman, L., "Study: Sexually Active Species More Immune to Disease," *Philadelphia Daily News,* November 2000, p. 46.

Broadhurst, L. C., "Phytochemicals: The Ties That Bind," *Nutrition Science News,* Boulder, CO, Vol. 6, No. 7, July 2001, pp. 262–64.

Brody, J. E., "Do You Need the Hormone of Desire?" *New York Times,* February 24, 1998.

Bucco, G., "Wild Yam for Menopause" *Let's Live,* Los Angeles, CA, Vol. 66, No. 1, January 1998, pp. 78–81.

Buckle, R., and Feliciano, J., "Supplemental Sex," *Muscle and Fitness,* Woodland Hills, CA, Vol. 5, No. 6, June 1997, pp. 148–50.

Butler, R., and Lewis, M., *Love and Sex After 60,* New York: Ballantine, 1993.

Carries, P., *Sexual Addition,* Minneapolis, MN: Compcare Publications, 1983.

Challem, J., "Chemical Warfare," *Prime Health and Fitness,* Woodland Hills, CA, Vol. 11, No. 4, Winter 1996, pp. 59–64.

Challem, J., "Prescription for Disaster," *Let's Live,* Los Angeles, CA, Vol. 68, No. 1, January 2000, pp. 46–49.

Challem, J., "St. John's Wort vs. Drugs," *Nutrition Science News,* Vol. 6, No. 6, June 2001, pp. 212–16.

Cheney, D. L., ed., *Monitoring Fluid and Electrolytes Precisely,* Horsham, PA: Eugene W. Jackson Publishing, 1979.

Cheraskin, E., Ringsdorf, W. M., and Brecher, A., *Psychodietetics,* New York: Bantam Books, 1974.

Cheung, T., *Androgen Disorders in Women,* Alameda, CA: Hunter House, 1999.

Chia, M., and Abrams, D., *The Multi-Orgasmic Man,* New York: HarperCollins, 1997.

Cichoke, A., *The Complete Book of Enzyme Therapy,* New York: Avery, 1999.

Claes, H., and Baert, I., "Pelvic Floor Exercises Versus Surgery in the Treatment of Impotence," *British Journal of Urology,* 1993, 71 (1): 52–57.

Claffin, E., ed., *The Female Body: An Owner's Manual,* Emmaus, PA: Rodale Press, 1995.

Coleman, D., "Death of a Sex Life" *Health,* Vol. 22, No. 4, April 1990, pp. 53–54.

Colker, C. M., *Sex Pills, Androstenedione to Zinc,* Hauppauge, NY: Advanced Research Press, 1999.

Colon, A. B., "Nature's Fire Starters," *Fitness Plus Magazine* Vol. 9, No. 7, July 1998, pp. 58–61.

Comfort, A., *More Joy: A Lovemaking Companion to The Joy of Sex,* New York: Crown Publishers, 1974.

Comfort, A., *The Joy of Sex,* New York: Crown, 1972, 1991.

Cooper, K. H., *The New Aerobics,* New York: M. Evans and Co. Inc., 1970.

Cooper, R. K., *High Energy Living,* Emmaus, PA: Rodale Press, 2000.

Corio, L. E., *The Change Before the Change,* New York: Bantam Books, 2000.

Cowley, G., "Attention Aging Men, Testosterone and Other Hormone Treatments Offer New Hope for Staying Youthful Sexy and Strong," *Newsweek*, September 1996, p. 68–75.

Cox, T., "Putting the OH in Orgasm," *Complete Woman*, Chicago, October/November 1999, pp. 41–43.

Crayhon, R., *Health Benfits of FOS (Fructooligosacharides)*, New Canaan, CT: Keats Publishing, 1995.

Credit, L. P., Hartunia, S. C., and Nowak, M. J., *Your Guide to Complementary Medicine*, Garden City Park NY: Avery, 1993.

Crenshaw, T. L., *The Alchemy of Love and Lust*, New York: G. P. Putnam's Sons, 1996.

Dager, S. R., et al., "Panic Disorder Precipitated by Exposure to Organic Solvents in Work Place," *American Journal of Psychiatry*, August 1987: 144: 1056–58.

Davis, J., *Endorphins*, Garden City, NY: Doubleday and Co., 1984.

Davis, L., "Shameless Sex," *Men's Health*, Rodale Press, Emmaus, PA, April 1995, pp. 108–11 and 130–31.

"DHEA Increases Well Being and Sex Drive In Women," *Let's Live*, Los Angeles, CA, Vol. 68, No. 1, January 2000, p. 22.

Diamond, J., *Male Menopause*, Naperville, IL: Source Books, Inc., 1997.

Ditzen, L. S., "U.S. Judge Approves Diet Drug Settlement," *Philadelphia Inquirer*, August 29, 2000, p. A1.

Dixon, A. F., "The Neuroendocrine Regulation of Sexual Behavior in Female Primates," *Annual Review of Sex Research*, 1990: (1) 197–226.

Dodson, B., *Sex for One: The Joy of Self-Loving*, New York: Harmony Books, 1987.

Dolby, V., "Nature's Aphrodisiacs," *Let's Live*, Los Angeles, CA, Vol. 66, No. 2, February 1998, pp. 66–71.

d'Raye, T., *The Oxygen Answer for Health and Healing*, Keizer, OR: Awicca Publishing, 1999.

Drug Store News, "OTC's Preferred Over Doctor's Visit, Study Finds," New York, April 23, 2001, p. 27.

Eagan, J., "On Matters of Sex," *Muscle Magazine International,* Hollywood, FL, December 2000, pp. 210–216.

Eagan, J., "On Matters of Sex, Sensual Foot Massages, Tongue Tied and Flying Solo," *Muscle Magazine International,* No. 220, October 2000, pp. 196–99.

Eisenberg, D. M. et al., "Trends in Alternative Medicine Use in the United States," *Journal of the American Medical Association,* November 11, 1998.

Eisenberg, D. M. et al., "Unconventional Medicine in the United States," *New England Journal of Medicine,* 1993: 328: 246–52.

Elliott, M., "How to Increase Your Supply of Growth Hormone," *Let's Live,* Los Angeles, CA, Vol. 68, No. 10, October 2000, pp. 52–54.

Erikson, E., *Identity: Youth and Crisis,* New York: W. W. Norton, 1968.

Erikson, E., *The Life Cycle Completed: A Review,* New York: W. W. Norton, 1982.

Faelten, S. (ed), *Natural Prescriptions for Women,* Emmaus, PA: Rodale Press, 1998.

Fallon, A., "Culture in the Mirror: Sociocultural Determinants of Body Image," in T. F. Cash and T. Pruzinskiy (eds), *Body Images: Development, Deviance and Change,* New York: Guilford Press, 1990, pp. 80–99.

Feldman, E. B., *Nutrition in the Middle and Later Years,* New York: Warner Books, 1986, p. 2.

Fernstrom, J. D., "Dietary Amino Acids and Brain Function," *Journal of the American Dietetic Association,* January 1994: 94(1): 71–77.

Ferrni, R., and Connor, E. B., "Caffeine Intake and Endogenous Sex Steroid Levels in Postmenopausal Women," *American Journal of Epidemiology,* 1994: 55(9): 406–13.

Fiedler, C., "Spring Cleaning," *Energy Times Magazine,* Long Beach, CA, Vol. 10, No. 6, June 2000, pp. 52–57.

Fisher, S., *The Female Orgasm,* New York: Basic Books, 1973.

Foster, S., *101 Medicinal Herbs,* Loveland, CO: Interweave Press, 1998.

Frank, E., "Frequency of Sexual Dysfunction in Normal Couples," *New England Journal of Medicine,* Vol. 299, 1978: 111–15.

Fredricks, C., *Carlton Fredericks' Nutritional Guide for the Prevention and Cure of Common Ailments and Diseases,* New York: Simon & Schuster, 1982.

Fried, R., and Merrell, W.C., *The Arginine Solution,* New York: Warner Books, 1999.

Freidman, L., et al., "Testicular Atrophy and Impaired Spermatogenesis in Rats Fed High Levels of the Methylxanthines Caffeine, Theobromine, Ortheophylline." *Journal of Environmental Pathology and Toxicology,* January–February 1979: 2: 687–706.

Fry, K., and Wingo, C., *Menopause Naturally,* Green Bay, WI: Impak Communications, 2000.

Gambrelli, R. D., Bagnell, C. A., and Greenblatt, R. B., "Role of Estrogens and Progesterone in the Etiology and Prevention of Endometrial Cancer: A Review," *American Journal of Obstetrics and Gynecology,* 1983 (146).

Garrison, R., and Somer, E., *The Nutrition Desk Reference,* New Canaan, CT: Keats Publishing, 1995.

Gelbard, M. K., *Solving Prostate Problems,* New York: Simon & Schuster, 1995.

Gelfand, M., "Estrogen-Androgen Hormone Replacement Therapy," *European Medical Journal,* 1995: 2(3): 22–26.

Gerber, M., "Chelation: The Love Therapy," *Alternative Medicine Digest,* No. 34, March 2000, pp. 58–60.

Gerber, M., "Maca Mania," *Alternative Medicine Digest,* No. 38, November 2000, pp.100–3.

Gerber, M., "Reich and Roll," *Alternative Medicine Digest,* No. 36, July 2000, pp. 98–102.

Gerber, M., "Stress: Adrenal Glands and Sex Responsiveness," *Alternative Medicine Digest,* No. 33, January 2000, pp. 66–68.

Gerlin, A., "Rooting Out Mistakes in Medicine," *Philadelphia Inquirer*, No. 254, Jan. 9, 2001, p. A1.

Gershon, L., *Growing Younger: Nutritional Rejuvenation for People Over Forty*, Los Angeles, CA: Tarcher/St. Martin's Press, 1987.

Geslewitz, C., "Sex Sells: Viagra Heats Up Market for Sexual Supplements," *Health Food Business*, Vol. 44, No. 12, Melville, NY, December 1998, pp. 36–39.

Gibson, R. A., and Kneebone, G. M., "Fatty Acid Composition of Human Colostrum and Mature Breast Milk," *American Journal of Clinical Nutrition*, 34 (1981): 252–57.

Gilbaugh, J. H., *A Doctor's Guide to Men's Private Parts*, New York: Crown, 1989.

Gilbert, M., "Managing Stress: Pathways to Adaptation and Balance," *Healthwell.com*, May 2001 (Copyright 2001 Penton Media, NC).

Girdano, D. A., Everly, G. S., and Dusek, D. E., *Controlling Stress and Tension: A Holistic Approach*, Englewood Cliffs, NJ: Prentice-Hall, 1990.

Glant, A., Zinner, S., and McCormick, W., "The Prevalence of Dyspareunia," *American Journal of Obstetries and Gynecology*, March 1996, Vol. 75, No. 3, pp. 433–36.

Goldberg, B., "Resisting Antibiotics," *Alternative Medicine Digest*, No. 26, October/November 1998, pp. 12–13.

Goldberg, B., "What We Must Do to Survive the 21st Century," *Alternative Medicine Digest*, January 2000, p. 8.

Goldberg, K. A., et al. (eds), *The Complete Book of Men's Health*. Emmaus, PA: Rodale Press, 1999.

Goldberg, L., and Elliot, D. L., *The Healing Power of Exercise*, New York: John Wiley, 2000.

Goldin, B. R., et al., "The Effects of Dietary Fat and Fiber on Serum Estrogen Concentrations in Premenopausal Women Under Controlled Dietary Conditions," *Cancer*, 1994 74(3): 1125–31.

Goldstein, I., and Berman, J. R., "Vasculogenic Female Sexual Dysfunction: Vaginal Engorgement and Clitoral Erectile Insufficiency," *International Journal of Impotence Research*, 1998: 10 (2): 84–90.

Goldstein, M., "Mediterranean Diet and Coronary Heart Disease," *Lancet,* July 1995, 344:276.

Gormley, J. J., Chronological Age Is Irrelevant If You Maintain a Healthful Lifestyle, *Better Nutrition,* Vol. 58, No. 4, April 1996, pp. 28–30.

Gots, R. E., *Chemical Sensitivity: The Truth About Environmental Illness*, Amherst, NY: Prometheus Books, 1998.

Goulant, S., "Are You Sexually Fit?" *Let's Live,* Los Angeles, CA, Vol. 64, No. 2, February 1996, pp. 38–42.

Gould, L. A., "Impact of Cardiovascular Disease on Male Sexual Function," *Medical Aspects of Human Sexuality*, Vol. 23, April 1989, 24–27.

Gould, R. L., *Transformations: Growth and Change in Adult Life,* New York: Simon & Schuster, 1978.

Graber, G. K., and Graber, B., *Woman's Orgasm,* New York: Warner Books, 1975.

Graham, J., *Evening Primrose Oil,* New York: Thorsons Publishers, 1984.

Granato, H., "Age of the Individual-Biochemical Individuality for Longer Life," *Health Supplement Retailer,* Phoenix, AZ, Vol. 7, No. 8, pp. 10–17.

Grandhi, A., Mujumdar, A. M., and Wardhan, P., "Comparative Pharmacological Investigation of Ashwagandlha and Ginseng," *Journal of Ethnopharmacology,* 1994: 44:131–35.

Grant, B., "You Are What You Eat: The Food Sex Connection," *Energy Times,* Vol. 4, No. 3, May/June 1994, pp. 21–26.

Gray, A., Feldman, H. A., McKinlay, J. B., et al., "Age Disease and Changing Sex Hormone Levels in Middle Aged Study," *Journal of Clinical Endocrinolic Metabolism,* 1991: 73: 1016–25.

Green, R, *Human Sexuality: A Health Practitioner's Text,* 2nd ed., Baltimore, MD: Williams and Wilkins, 1979.

Groggains, J., *Fit Happens*, New York: Villard, 2000.

Guyton, A. C., *Function of the Human Body*, 3rd ed., Philadelphia, PA: W. B. Saunders, 1969.

Haas, E., "Transform Your Health With the Detox Diet," *Natural Remedies*, Stamford, CT, October 1997, pp 64–69.

Hallfrisca, J., et al. "High Plasma Vitamin C Associated With High Plasma HDL2 Cholesterol," *American Journal of Clinical Nutrition*, 1994: 60: 100–5.

Hammond, D. B., *My Parents Never Had Sex: Myths and Facts of Sexual Aging*, Buffalo, NY: Prometheus Books, 1985.

Hanson, C., *Grape Seed Extract*, New York: Healing Wisdom Publications, 1995.

Hanson, P. G., *The Joy of Stress*, Kansas City, MO: Andrews McMeel and Parker, 1985.

Harriman, S., *The Book of Ginseng*, New York: Jove Pubications, 1973.

Hass, R., *Eat Smart, Think Smart*, New York: HarperCollins, 1994.

Hassam, A. G., Sinclair, A. J., and Crawford, M. A., "The Incorporation of Orally Fed Radioactive Gammalinolenic Acid and Linoleic Acid into the Liver and Brain Lipids of Suckling Rats," *Lipids* 7 (1995): 417–420.

Haynes, K., "The O Zone," *Natural Remedies*, Oak Park, IL, March/April 1998, pp. 42–45.

Henderson, D. R., and Mitchell, D., *Colostrum: Nature's Healing Miracle*, Salt Lake City, UT: CNR Publications, 1999.

Hendler, S. S. *The Complete Guide to Anti-Aging Nutrients*, New York: Simon & Schuster, 1985.

Hendrix, H., *Getting the Love You Want: A Guide for Couples*, New York: Harper and Row, 1990.

Henry, J. P., "Biological Basis of the Stress Response," *Integrative Physiology of Behavioral Science*, 1992, 27(1), 66–83.

Herbal Research Publications, *Naturopathic Handbook of Herbal Formulas*, Ayer, MA: Herbal Research Publications Inc., 1995.

Hill, H. E., *Introduction to Lecithin*, New York: Nash Publishing, 1972.

Hite, S., *The Hite Report on Male Sexuality*, New York: Ballantine, 1981.

Hobbs, C., *Stress and Natural Healing*, Loveland, CO: Interweave Press, 1997.

Hobbs, C., "Using Herbs: A Practical Guide," *Let's Live*, Los Angeles, CA, Vol. 62, No. 12, December 1994, pp.16–20.

Hofmekler, O., "Fats That Heal, Fats That Kill: An Exclusive Interview With Fat Guru Udo Erasmus," *Mind and Muscle Power*, Vol. 1, No. 1, January 2000, pp. 56–57.

Hollander, E., and McCarley, A., "Yohimbine Treatment of Sexual Side Effects Induced by Serotonin Reuptake Blockers," *Journal of Clinical Psychiatry*, 1992: 53(6): 207–9.

Holt, S., *The Sexual Revolution*, San Diego, CA: Promotional Publishing, 1999.

Howell, E., *Enzyme Nutrition: The Food Enzyme Concept*, Garden City Park, NY: Avery, 1985.

Hrachovec, J. P., *Keeping Young and Living Longer*, Los Angeles, CA: Sherbourne Press, 1972.

Hunter, B. T., *Food Additives and Federal Policy: The Mirage of Safety*, New York: Charles Scribner's Sons, 1975.

James, S. H., and Grace, W., "Life Stress and Cancer of the Cervix," *Psychosomatic Medicine*, Vol. 16, No. 4, 1954 (4): 287–94.

Jarow, J., Kloner, R. A., and Holmes, A. M., *Viagra*, New York: M. Evans and Co., 1998.

Jarry, H., Harnischfeger, G., and Duker, E., "Study on the Endocrine Efficacy of the Constituents of Cimicifuga Recemosa," *Plant Medica*, 1985: 51(4): 316–19.

Jensen, B., and Bell, S., *Tissue Cleansing Through Bowel Management*, Escondido, CA: Bernard Jensen International, 1981.

Johanson, S., *Sex Is Perfectly Natural, but Not Naturally Perfect*, New York: Penguin Books, 1991.

Johnson, D. W., and Mokler, D. J., "Lecithin's Therapeutic Effects," *New Hope Institute of Retailing*, June 2001, pp. 1–8.

Johnson, L., "Spring Cleansing," *Herbs for Health*, Golden Co., Vol. 3, No. 1, pp. 28–33.

Johnson, M., "OTC's Preferred Over Doctor's Visit, Study Finds," *OTC/Natural Health, Drug Store News*, April 23, 2001, p. 27.

Jones, S. S., "Superfoods: Eating Greens for Radiant Health," *Let's Live*, Los Angeles, CA, Vol. 62, No. 12, December 1994, pp. 32–37.

Joyal, S., "Jumpstart Your Anabolic Drive: The Dopamine Connection," *Mind and Muscle Power*, Vol. 1, No. 8, November 2000, pp. 38–41.

Kaiser, F., et al., "Impotence and Aging: Clinical and Hormonal Factors," *Journal of the American Geriatric Society*, 1988, 36: 511–19.

Kalman, D., "Mind Power: Feed Your Head," *Mind and Muscle Power*, Vol. 1, No. 1, January 2000, pp. 77–79.

Kalman, D. S., "Branched Chain Amino Acids," *Physical*, Los Angeles, CA, Vol. 3, No. 3, March 2000, pp. 55–57.

Kapatos, G., and Zigmond, M. "Dopamine Biosynthesis From L. Tyrosine and L. Phenylalanine in Rat Brain Synaptosomes: Preferential Use of Newly Accumulated Precursons," *Journal of Neurochemistry*, May 1977: (5):1109–19.

Kaplan, H., and Owen, T., "The Female Androgen Deficiency Syndrome," *Journal of Sex and Marital Therapy*, 1993: 19 (1): 3–24.

Kaplan, H. S., *Disorders of Sexual Desire and Other New Concepts and Techniques in Sex Therapy*, New York: Bruner/Mazel, 1979.

Kaplan, H. S., *The New Sex Therapy*, New York: Bruner/Mazel, 1974.

Katzenstein, L., and Katlowitz, N., *Viagra: The Potency Promise*, New York: St. Martin's Press, 1998.

Kaunitz, A., "The Role of Androgens in Menopausal Hormonal Replacement," *Menopause and Hormone Replacement Therapy*, 1997: 26 (2): 391–97.

Keesling, B., *All Night Long: How to Make Love to a Man Over 50*, New York: HarperCollins, 2000.

Keesling, B., *Getting Close: A Lover's Guide to Embracing Fantasy and Heightening Sexual Connection*, New York: HarperCollins, 1999.

Keesling, B., *How to Make Love All Night (and Drive a Woman Wild)*, New York: HarperPerennial, 1994.

Keesling, B., *Sexual Pleasure*, Alameda, CA: Hunter House, 1993.

Kegel, A. H., "Sexual Functions and the Pubbosccygeus Muscle," *Western Journal of Surgery*, 60 (1952): 521–24.

Khalsa, K. P. S., "Peruvian Sex Herb and More MACA," *Let's Live*, Los Angeles, CA, Vol. 67, No. 11, November 1999, pp. 49–51.

Khurana, R. C., *You and Your Hormone Glands*, Pittsburgh, PA: Obesity and Diabetes Books Publishing, 1978.

Kilham, C., "Stalking the Rain Forest Viagra," *Let's Live*, Los Angeles, CA, Vol. 67, No. 9, September 1999, pp. 53–54.

Kilham, C., "The New Sex Potion: Can It Change Your Life on the Medicine Trail in Search of Horny Goat Weed," Hicksville, NY: Bodyonics LTD, 2001.

Kilmann, P. R., and Mills, K. H., *All About Sex Therapy*, New York: Plenum Press, 1983.

Kinsey, A., *Sexual Behaviors in the Human Female*, Philadelphia: W. B. Saunders, 1953.

Kinsey, A., *Sexual Behaviors in the Human Male*, Philadelphia: W. B. Saunders, 1948.

Kinsey, A. C., Pomeroy, W. B., Martin, C. E., and Gebhard, P. H. *Sexual Behavior in the Human Female*, Philadelphia: W. B. Saunders, 1966.

Kinsey, A. C., Pomeroy, W. B., Martin, C. E., and Gebhard, P. H. *Sexual Behavior in the Human Male*, Philadelphia, PA: W. B. Saunders, 1966.

Klatz, R., *Growing Young With HGH*, New York: HarperPerennial, 1997.

Kleiner, S. M., *High Performance Nutrition*, New York: John Wiley, 1996.

Kloner, A., and Zusman R. M., "Cardiovascular Effects of Sildenafil

Citrate and Recommendations for Its Use," *American Journal of Cardiology*, Vol. 84, No. 5B, pp. 11N–17N.

Kloss, J., *Back to Eden*, Twin Lakes, WI: Lotus Press Co., 1997.

Kluger, J., "Can We Stay Young?" *Time Magazine*, Vol. 148, No. 24, pp. 88–98.

Knox, A., "Glaxo Takes Drug Off Market," *Philadelphia Inquirer*, November 29, 2001, p. C1.

Knox, A., "New Drugs Bringing More Risk and Recalls," *Philadelphia Inquirer*, February 7, 2001, p. 1.

Kobayashi, Y., "Pheromones: The Smell of Beauty," International English Center, University of Colorado, December 16, 1997, online at: The Pheromone News: http//:www.pheromones.com.

Kohl, J., *The Secret of Eros: Mysteries of Odor in Human Sexuality*, online at: http//:www.pheromones.com.

Kressler, R., "Complications of Inflatable Penile Prostheses," *Urology*, 1981 (18): 470–73.

Ladis, A., Whipple, B., and Perry, J., *The G-Spot and Other Recent Discoveries About Human Sexuality*, New York: Holt, Rinehart and Winston, 1982.

Lafavore, M. (ed), *Men's Health Advisor 1995*, Emmaus, PA: Rodale Press, 1995.

Lafavore, M. (ed), *Men's Health Advisor 1993*, Emmaus, PA: Rodale Press, 1993.

Landis, R., and Khalsa, R.S., *Herbal Defense*, New York: Warner Books, 1997.

Lane, J., "Oil Change," *Energy Times Magazine*, Long Beach, CA, Vol. 9, No. 10, November/December 1999, pp. 61–68.

Lark, S., *The Menopause Self-Help Book: A Women's Guide to Feeling Good All Month*, Berkeley, CA: Celestial Arts, 1993.

Laucella, L., *Hormone Replacement Therapy: Conventional Medicine and Natural Alternatives*, Los Angeles, CA: Lowell House, 1999.

Lauersen, N., and Whitney, S., *It's Your Body: A Woman's Guide to Gynecology,* New York: Berkley Publishing, 1983.

Laumann, E. O., Park, A., and Rosen R. C., "Sexual Dysfunction in the United States: Prevalence and Predictors," *Journal of the American Medical Association,* 281 (1999): 537–44.

Lee, J. R., *What Your Doctor May Not Tell You About Menopause,* New York: Warner Books, 1996.

Lee, V., *Soulful Sex,* Berkeley, CA: Conari Press, 1996.

Lee, W. H, *Chorella,* New Canaan, CT: Keats Publishing, 1987.

Lee, W.H., *Pre-Menstrual Syndrome,* New Canaan, CT: Keats Publishing, 1984.

Lee, W. H., *Amazing Amino Acids,* New Canaan, CT: Keats Publishing, 1984.

Lee, W. H., *Bee Pollen: Super Energy—Super Nutrition,* New Canaan, CT: Keats Publishing, 1983.

LeGal, M., Cathebras, P., and Strawberry, K., "Pharmaton Capsules in the Treatment of Functional Fatigue: A Double Blind Study Versus Placebo Evaluated by a New Methodology," *Phytotherapy Research,* 1996, 10(1): 49–53.

Leibovitz, B., *Carnitine: The Vitamin BT Phenomenon,* New York: Dell Publications, 1984.

Leland, J., "A Pill for Impotence?" *Newsweek,* November 17, 1997, pp. 62–68.

Levine, R. A., *Culture, Behavior and Personality,* New York: Aldine Publishers, 1979.

Levins, H., *American Sex Machines,* Holbrook, MA: Adams Media, 1996.

Leviton, R., "Problem Free Erections," *Alternative Medicine Digest,* Tiburon, CA, No. 28, March 1999, pp. 40–45.

Ley, B. M., "DHEA: Miracle or Medicine?" *Prime Health and Fitness,* Woodland Hills, CA, Vol. 11, No. 4, Winter 1996, pp. 66–68.

Libby, R., "Prime Time Sex," *Journal of Longevity Research,* Vol. 2, No. 6, 1996: 13–14.

Libby, R., "Take Care of Your Sexual Health," *The Doctor's Prescription for Healthy Living,* Wilmington, DE, Vol. 2, No. 4, 1998, p. 4.

Liberman, S., and Bruning, N., *Design Your Own Vitamin and Mineral Program,* Garden City Park, NY: Doubleday, 1987.

Liberman, S., and Bruning, N., *The Real Vitamin and Mineral Book,* Garden City Park, NY: Avery, 1997.

Lieblum, S., "Vaginal Atrophy of the Postmenopausal Women," *Journal of the American Medical Association,* 1983, Vol. 249, No. 16.

Liebowitz, M. R., *The Chemistry of Love,* Boston, MA: Little, Brown, 1983.

Lipkiss, A., "Carnosine a Protective Anti-Aging Peptide," *International Journal of Biochemistry and Cell Biology,* 1998, 30: S63–S68.

Lloyd, J. E., *Nice Couples Do: How to Turn Your Secret Dreams Into Sensational Sex,* New York: Warner Books, 1991.

Longgood, W., *The Poisons in Your Food,* New York: Pyramid Books, 1969.

Lynch, J., *The Broken Heart: The Medical Consequences of Loneliness,* New York: Basic Books, 1979.

Mackarness, R., *Living Safely in a Polluted World,* New York: Stein and Day, 1980.

Maher, T., "L-Arginine," *New Hope Institute of Retailing (Continuing Education Modules),* Boulder, CO, February 2000.

Maheux, R., Naud, F., Rioux, M., et al., "A Randomized Double-Blind, Placebo-Controlled Study on the Effects of Conjugated Estrogen on Skin Thickness." *American Journal of Obstetrics and Gynecology,* 1994 170: 642.

Mangolies, E., *Undressing the American Male: Men With Sexual Problems and What Women Can Do to Help Them,* New York: Penguin Books, 1994.

Masters, W. H., Johnson, V., and Kolodny, R. C., *Heterosexuality,* New York: HarperCollins, 1994.

Masters, W. H., and Johnson, V. E., *Human Sexual Inadequacy,* Boston: Little, Brown and Company, 1970.

Masters, W.H., and Johnson, V., *Human Sexual Response,* Boston: Little, Brown and Company, 1966.

Mathis, S., "How to Increase Your Supply of Growth Hormone," *Let's Live,* Los Angeles, CA, Vol. 67, No. 9, September 1999, pp. 61–62.

Marin, P., et al., "Adrogen Treatment of Middle Aged Obese Men: Effects on Metabolism, Muscle and Adipose Tissue," *European Medicine* (1992): 1 (6): 329–36.

Marsa, L., "Medical Studies Call for Some Healthy Scepticism," *Philadelphia Inquirer,* May 14, 2001, p. D1.

Marshal, L. A., "Velvet Antler Under the Microscope," *Nutrition Science News,* Boulder, CO, Vol. 5, No. 3, March 2000, pp.104–6, 132.

Martlew, G., *Electrolyes the Spark of Life,* Murdock, FL: Nature's Publishing, 1994.

Martinez, B., and Staba, J., "The Physiological Effect of Panax and Eleuthreroccocus on Exercised Rats," *Japanese Journal of Pharmacology,* 1984: 35(2): 79–85.

Mayell, M., *Natural Energy: A Consumer's Guide to Legal, Mind-Altering and Mood-Brightening Herbs and Supplements,* New York: Three Rivers Press, 1998.

McCary, J. L., *McCary's Human Sexuality,* 3rd ed., New York: Van Nostrand Reinhold, 1978.

McDougall, C., "High Voltage Sex: Joy Buzzers," *Men's Health,* June 1990, pp. 70–71.

McIlvenna R. L., *The Pleasure Quest: The Search for Aphrodisiacs,* San Francisco: The Institute for Advanced Study of Human Sexuality, 1988, p. 11.

McQuade, W., and Aikman, A., *Stress,* New York: E. P. Dutton and Co., 1974.

Memmler, R. L., Cohen, B. J., and Wood, D. L., *The Human Body in Health and Disease,* 7th ed., New York: J. B. Lippincott, 1992.

Miller, H. I., "Still Hazardous to Your Health," *Consumers Research,* Washington, D.C., Vol. 8, No. 1, pp. 10, 13–16.

Milsten R., and Slowinski, J., *The Sexual Male: Problem and Solutions,* New York: W.W. Norton and Co., 1999.

Mindell, E., *Earl Mindell's Herb Bible,* New York: Simon & Schuster, 1992.

Mittleman, M. A., et al., "Incidence of Myocardial Infarction and Death in 53 Clinical Trials of Viagra (Sildenafil Citrate)," *American College of Cardiologist Conference Abstracts,* Vol. 35, No. 2, Suppl. A, February 2000, p. 302.

Mobley, D. F., and Wilson, S. K., *Reversing Impotence Forever!* Alvin, TX: Swan Publishing, 1995.

Moglia, R. F., and Knowles, J., *All About Sex: A Family Resource on Sex and Sexuality,* New York: Three Rivers Press, 1993.

Morgan, B. L. C., and Morgan, R., *Hormones,* Los Angeles, CA: The Body Press, 1989.

Moore, L., "Male Potency: Strategies for Getting a Rise Out of Your Sex Life, *Mind and Muscle Power,* New York, Vol. 1, January 2000, pp. 34–36.

Moore, L. M., "Oxytocin Stimulates Anabolic Hormone Released in Orgasms and Mother's Milk," *Mind and Muscle Power,* New York, Vol. 1, No. 8, November 2000, pp. 20–23.

Morter, M. T., *Your Health, Your Choice,* Hollywood, FL: Lifetime Books, 1993.

Mowrey, D., "Get Moving," *Energy Times,* Long Beach, CA, January 1996, pp. 50–56.

Murray, M., *Dr. Murray's Total Body Tune-Up,* New York: Bantam Books, 2000.

Murray, M., and Pizzorno, J., *Encyclopedia of Natural Medicine,* Rocklin, CA: Prima Publishing, 1997.

Murray, M. T., "Natural Alternatives to Viagra," *Let's Live,* Los Angeles, CA, August 1998, pp. 46–49.

Muryn, M., *Water Magic: Healing Bath Recipes for the Body, Spirit and Soul,* New York: Simon & Schuster, 1995.

Nabulsi, A. A., et al., "Association of Hormone-Replacement Therapy With Various Cardiovascular Risk Factors in Postmenopausal Women," *New England Journal of Medicine,* 1993: 328: 1069–75.

Nachtigall, L., and Heilman, J. R., *Estrogen,* New York: Harper and Row, 1986.

Naguib, Y., "OPC Antioxidant Superstar," *Vitamin Retailer,* East Brunswick, NJ, Vol. 8, No. 2, February 2001, pp. 38–41.

Niels, L., and Whitney, S., *It's Your Body: A Woman's Guide to Gynecology,* New York: Grosset & Dunlap Inc., 1983.

Norman, K., "Nutrition Is the Keystone of Prevention," *American Journal of Clinical Nutrition,* 1994: 60:1.

Northrup, C., *Women's Bodies, Women's Wisdom,* New York: Bantam Books, 1989.

Notelovitz, M., and Tonnessien, D., *Menopause and Midlife Health,* New York: St. Martin's Press, 1993.

Offit, A. K., *The Sexual Self,* Philadelphia: J. B. Lippincott Co., 1977.

Ogden, G., *Women Who Love Sex,* New York: Pocket Books, 1994.

Ojeda, L., *Menopause Without Medicine,* Alameda, CA: Hunter House, 1989.

Orentreich, N., Brind, J., et al., "Age Changes and Sex Differences in Serum Dehydroepiandrosterone Sulfate Concentrations Throughout Adulthood," *Journal of Clinical Encrinology Metabolism,* 59(3): 1984, 557–64.

Orey, C., "20 Ways to Get Him to Notice You," *Complete Woman,* Chicago, IL, October/November 1999, pp. 12–13, 76.

Orey, C., "Virility/Femininity Quest," *Energy Times,* Long Beach, CA, Vol. 10, No. 2, February 2000, pp. 38–41.

Ornstein, R., and Sobel, D., *Healthy Pleasures,* Reading, MA: Addison Wesley, 1989.

Padus, E., *The Complete Guide to Your Emotions and Your Health,* Emmaus, PA: Rodale Press, 1986.

Padus, E., *The Woman's Encyclopedia of Health and Natural Healing,* Emmaus, PA: Rodale Press, 1981.

Palmore, E. B., "Predictors of the Longevity Difference: A 25-Year Follow-Up." *Gerontolgist,* 6 (1982): 513–18.

Passwater, R., *Spirulina,* New Canaan, CT: Keats Publishing, 1981.

Pauling, L., *How to Live Longer and Feel Better,* New York: W. H. Freeman and Co., 1986.

Pearsall, P., *Sexual Healing,* New York: Crown, 1994.

Pearsall, P., *Super Marital Sex: Loving for Life,* New York: Doubleday, 1987.

Pearsall, P., "Use It or Lose It," *Living Fit,* Woodland Hills, CA, January/ February 1996, pp. 188–89.

Pearson, D., and Shaw, S., *Life Extension.* New York: Warner Books, 1982.

Pearlstein, T., "Hormones and Depression: What Are the Facts About Premenstrual Syndrome Menopause and Hormone Replacement Therapy," *American Journal of Obstetrics and Gynecology* 1995. 173: 646–653.

Peiper, H., and Anderson, N., *Natural Solutions for Sexual Dysfunction,* East Canaan, CT: Safe Goods, 1998.

Pelletier, K. L., *Longevity: Fulfilling Our Biological Potential,* New York: Delacorte Publishing, 1984.

Penney, A., *How to Make Love to a Man,* New York: Dell, 1990.

Perlmutter, D., "Adverse Drug Reactions: A Major Cause of Death," *Perlmutter Letter,* Naples, FL, Vol. 4, No. 1, Summer 1998, p. 2.

Perlmutter, D., "Pharmaceutical Drugs: A Prescription for Danger," *The Perlmutter Letter,* Naples, FL, Vol. 4, No. 2, Summer 1998, p. 1.

Perper, T., *Sex Signals: The Biology of Love,* Philadelphia, PA: ISI Press, 1981.

Perry, S., and O'Hanlan, K., *Natural Menopause,* Reading, MA: Addison Wesley, 1992.

Phillips, D., and Judd, R., *Sexual Confidence: Discovering the Joy of Intimacy,* Boston: Houghton Mifflin, 1980.

Phillips, L., "Ask Yourself This: Is He Your Sexual Soul-Mate?" *Complete Woman,* Chicago, October/November 1999, pp. 6–8.

Pierpaoli, W., Regelson, W., and Colman, C., *The Melatonin Miracle,* New York: Simon & Schuster, 1995.

Pike, A., *Nutrition Benefits of Oyster Extract,* Kuze Minami-ku, Kyoto: Sagawa Publishers Co. Ltd., 1980.

Poppy, J., "The Big Bang: If Women Can Have Incredible Earth Shaking Orgasms, Why Can't You?" *Men's Health,* Emmaus, PA., Vol. 10, No. 5, June 1995, pp. 122–24.

Poticha, J., *Use It or Lose It,* New York: Richard Markek Publishers, 1978.

Potter, S., Baum, J., Honguy, T., Rachel, J., et al., "Soy Proteins and Isoflavones: Their Effects on Blood Lipids and Bone Density in Postmenopausal Women," *American Journal of Clinical Nutrition,* 1998, 68: 1375S–79S.

Product Report, "Horny Goat Weed," *Vitamin Retailer,* East Brunswick, NJ, Vol. 8, No. 2, February 2001, p. 46.

Quilliam, S., *Every Woman's Guide to Sexual Fulfillment,* London: Marshall Edition, 1997.

Rajfer, J., et al., "Nitric Oxide as a Mediator of Relaxation of the Corpus Cavernosum in Response to Nonadrenergic, Noncholinergic, Neurotransmission," *New England Journal of Medicine,* 1992: 326 (2): 90–94.

Rako, S., *The Hormone of Desire: The Truth About Testosterone, Sexuality, and Menopause,* New York: Harmony Books, 1996.

Rath, M., *Why Animals Don't Get Heart Attacks but People Do,* Freemont, CA: Matthias Rath Inc., 1999.

Raymond, C., "Virile Without Viagra," *Natural Way Magazine,* Boulder, CO, Vol. 4. No. 4, September–October 1998, pp. 58–64.

Raymond, N., "Defend Your Liver," *Great Life*, Los Angeles, CA, Vol. 4, No. 7, July 2001, pp. 20–21.

Redmon, G., "Can Food Enhance Your Sex Drive," *Muscle and Fitness*, Woodland Hill, CA, Vol. 58, February 1997, pp. 132–34, 188.

Redmon, G., *Managing and Preventing Arthritis: The Natural Alternatives*, Prescott, AZ: Hohm Press, 1999.

Redmon, G., *Minerals: What Your Body Needs and Why*, Garden City Park, NY: Avery, 1999.

Redmon, G. L., *Energy for Life: How to Overcome Chronic Fatigue*, Bloomingdale, IL: Vital Health Publishing, 2000.

Redmon, G. L., *Managing and Preventing Prostate Disorders*, Prescott, AZ: Hohm Press, 2000.

Regelson, W., and Colman, C., *The Superhormone Promise*, New York: Simon & Schuster, 1996.

Reichman, J., *I'm Not in the Mood: What Every Woman Should Know About Improving Her Libido*, New York: William Morrow, 1998.

Renshaw, D., *Seven Weeks to Better Sex*, New York: Random House, 1995.

Reuben, D., *Everything You Always Wanted to Know About Sex: But Were Afraid to Ask*, New York: Bantam Books, 1969.

Reuters, P., "Study: Drug Aids Impotent," *Philadelphia Daily News*, January 2, 1997, p. 19.

Roberts, A., and Yawn, B. P., (eds), *Reader's Digest Guide to Love and Sex*, Pleasantville, NY: Reader's Digest, 1998.

Robinson, R., "Soy Foods Get Labeled," *Let's Live*, Los Angeles, CA, Vol. 67, No. 11, November 1999, pp. 83–85.

Rogers, S., *Chemical Sensitivity*, New Canaan, CT: Keats Publishing, 1995.

Roizen, M. F., *Real Age: Are You As Young As You Can Be?* New York: HarperCollins, 1999.

Romoff, A., *Estrogen: How and Why It Can Save Your Life*, New York: Golden Books, 1999.

Rorie, S., "The Art of Holistic Cleansing," *Health Supplement Retailer,* Phoenix, AZ, Vol. 7, No. 1, February 2001, pp. 31–33.

Rose, G., "Eat With Awareness," *Let's Live,* Los Angeles, CA, Vol. 62, No. 12, December 1994, pp. 24–27.

Rosenbaum, M. E., *The Amazing Superfood of the Orient,* Torrance, CA: Sun Wellness Inc., 1998.

Rosenik, "Great Greens," *Let's Live,* Vol. 67, No. 11, November 1999, pp. 44–47.

Roth, G., *When Food Is Love: Exploring the Relationship Between Eating and Intimacy,* New York: E. P. Dutton, 1992, p. 2.

Roth, G., and Watson, R. (eds), *The Medical Advisor: The Complete Guide to Alternative and Conventional Treatment,* Alexandria, VA: Time-Life Books, 1996.

Roughan, P. A., and Kunst, L., "Do Pelvic Floor Exercises Really Improve Orgasmic Potential?" *Journal of Sex and Marital Therapy* 7 (1981): 223–29.

Royal, P. C., *Herbally Yours,* Hurrican, UT: Sound Nutrition, 1994.

Ruben, J., "Beyond Probiotic," *Mind and Muscle Power,* New York, Vol. 1, No. 8, November 2000, p. 32.

Sahelian, R., *Melatonin: Nature's Sleeping Pill,* Marina Del Rey, CA: Be Happier Press, 1996.

Santillo, H., *Food Enzymes,* Prescott, AZ: Hohm Press, 1987.

Sare, C., "Water Shortage," *Muscle and Fitness,* Woodhills, CA: November 1998, pp. 220–22.

Schover, L. R., *Prime Time: Sexual Health for Men Over Fifty,* New York: Holt, Rinehart and Winston, 1984.

Seaman, B., and Seaman, G., *Women and the Crisis in Sex Hormones,* New York: Rawson Associates, 1977.

Sears, B., *Enter the Zone,* New York: Regan Books, 1995.

Selye, H., *The Stress of Life,* New York: McGraw-Hill, 1976.

Selye, H., *Stress Without Distress,* New York: Lippincott and Crowell, 1974.

Semans, J. H., "Premature Ejaculation: A New Approach," *Southern Medical Journal,* 49, 1956, pp. 353–58.

Serrett, A., Macciadl, F., Verga, M., et al., "Tyrosine Hydroxylase Gende Associated With Depressive Symptomatology in Mood Disorder," *American Journal of Genetics,* March 28, 1988, 81 (2): 127–30.

Shahani, K. M., and Ayebo, A. D., "Role of Dietary Lactobacilli in Gastro-Intestinal Microecology," *American Journal of Clinical Nutrition,* November 1980: 33:2445–57.

Sheehy, G., *The Silent Passage: Menopause,* New York: Pocket Books, 1993.

Shippen, E., *The Testosterone Syndrome,* New York: M. Evans and Co., 1998.

Shook, E. E., *Advanced Treatise in Herbology,* Beaumont, CA: Trinity Center Press, 1978.

Siegel, B. S., *Peace, Love and Healing,* New York: Harper and Row, 1989.

Siegel, M. E., *What Every Man Should Know About His Prostate,* New York: Walker and Co., 1988.

Silber, S., *The Male: From Infancy to Old Age,* New York: Charles Scribner's Sons, 1982.

Silver, H., *The Body-Smart System: The Complete Guide to Cleansing and Rejuvenation,* New York: Bantam Books, 1990.

Smith, G. D., Frankel, S., and Yannell, J., "Sex and Death: Are They Related? Findings from the Caerphilly Cohort Study," *British Medical Journal,* 315 (1997): 1641–44.

Smith, R., *The Dieter's Guide to Weight Loss During Sex,* New York: Workman Publishing, 1978.

Sobel, E., "The Wonderful Omega-3's and Other Good for You Fats," *Energy Times Magazine,* Vol. 10, No. 6, June 2000, pp. 58–62.

Soloman, N., *Liquid Island Noni (Morinda Citrifoloia),* Pleasant Grove, UT: Woodland Publishing, 1998.

Somer, E., *Food and Mood,* New York: Henry Holt, 1995.

Sparkman, D. S., "The Hormones That Control Growth: Testosterone— The King of Anabolic Hormones," *Muscular Development*, Ronkonkoma, NY, Vol. 33, No. 4, April 1996, pp. 169 and 188.

Stansbury, J. "A Well-Oiled Machine," *Nutrition Science News*, Boulder, CO, Vol. 5, No. 12, December 2000, pp. 502–5.

Stansbury, J., "Detox Therapies," *Health and Nutrition Breakthroughs*, Boulder, CO, Vol. 2, No. 5, May 1998, pp. 22–27.

Starr, B. D., and Weiner M. B., *The Starr-Weiner Report on Sex and Sexuality in the Mature Years*, New York: Stein and Day Publishers, 1981.

Steinberg, D. (ed), *Erotic by Nature: A Celebration of Life, of Love, and of Our Wonderful Bodies*, Santa Cruz, CA: Down There Press/Red Alden Books, 1988.

Subbiah, P. V., et al., "Effect of Dietary Supplementation With Marine Lipid Concentration on the Plasma Lipoprotein Composition of Hypercholesterolemic Patients," *Atherosclersosis*, October 1989, No. 2–3: 157–66.

Svitil, K., "Tired No More," *Vitamins Herbs and Health*, Vol. VIII, No. 4, 1998, pp. 24–26.

Tan, R. S., *The Andropause Mystery*, Houston, TX: Amred Publishing, 2001.

Taylor, K., "Woman's Word: Older Men Know What's Up: Getting to the Bottom of Why Sex Improves With Age," *Prime Health and Fitness*, Woodland Hills, CA, Vol. 11, No. 4, Winter 1996, p. 128.

Tennison, D. M., "Medicinal Teas for Women," *Let's Live*, Los Angeles, CA., Vol. 66, No. 2, February 1998, pp. 58–63.

The Boston Women's Health Book Collective, *Our Bodies, Ourselves*, New York: Simon & Schuster, 1998.

Tienna, L., *The Herbs of Life*, Freedom, CA: The Crossing Press, 1992.

Tilden, J. H., *Toxemia: The Basic Cause of Disease*, Chicago, IL: Natural Hygiene Press, 1974.

Tollision, R. D., "Speeding Drug Approvals, Safely, Privately," *Consumer's Research*, Washington, D.C., Vol. 81, No. 1, pp. 14–16.

Townsley, C., *Cleansing Made Simple*, Littleton, CO: LFH Publishing, 1997.

Trickey, R., *Women, Hormones and the Menstrual Cycle: Herbal and Medical Solutions from Adolescence to Menopause*, St. Leonards, Australia: Allen and Unwin, 1998.

Turner, L., "Boost Your Fertility," *Great Life*, Stamford, CT, February 2000, pp. 34–37.

Turner, L., "Sex and Food: Eating for Pleasure," *Healthy and Natural Journal*, Sarasota, FL, Vol. 6, No. 2, Issue 27, April 1999, pp. 34–35.

Turner, L., "Velvet Antler," *Vitamin Retailer*, East Brunswick, NJ, Vol. 7, No. 5, May 2000, pp. 42–49.

Turner, T., "Detoxify Your Body," *Let's Live*, Los Angeles, CA, Vol. 66, No. 1, January 1998, pp. 59–63.

Ulene, A., and Ulene, V., *The Vitamin Strategy*, Berkeley, CA: Ulysses Press, 1994.

University Medical Research Publishers, *Amazing Medicines the Drug Companies Don't Want You to Discover*, Tempe, AZ: 1993.

Ursell, A., *Complete Guide to Healing Foods*, New York: Dorling Kindersley, 2000.

Vaughan, D., "The Sex Pill Craze," *Your Health*, Boca Raton, FL, Vol. 37, No. 6, August 1998, pp. 50–52.

Viscott, D., *Emotionally Free: Letting Go of the Past to Live in the Moment*, Chicago, IL: 1993.

Vroon, P., *Smell: The Secret Seducer*, New York: Farrar, Straus and Giroux, 1994.

Wade, C., *Health Secrets From the Orient*, West Nyack, NY: Parker Publishing, 1973.

Wade, C., *Inner Cleansing*, Paramus, NJ: Prentice-Hall, 1992.

Walker, M., "Why Doctors of the Future Will Prescribe Whole Foods as Medicine," *Vita-Mix Special Report*, Cleveland, OH, February 1995, pp. 6–11.

Walker, N. M., *Fresh Vegetable and Fruit Juices*, Prescott, AZ: Norwalk Press, 1970.

Wallace, R. A., Biology, *The World of Life*, 5th Ed, Glenview, IL: Scott Foresman and Company, 1990.

Wallner, K., *Prostate Cancer: A Non-Surgical Perspective,* New York: Smart Medicine Press, 1996.

Walsh, P. C., and Worthington, J. F., *The Prostate: A Guide for Men and the Women Who Love Them,* Baltimore, MD: Johns Hopkins University Press, 1995.

Watson, C. M., "Better Sex at Midlife for Women," *Let's Live,* Los Angeles, CA, Vol. 68, No. 11, pp. 31–34.

Watson, C. M., *Love Potions,* Los Angeles, CA: Jeremy P. Tarcher, 1993.

Weber, C. A., "The New Sex Pill That Works," *Muscular Development,* Ronkonkoma, NY, Vol. 33, No. 4, April 1996, pp. 164–65.

Webster, D., *Acidophilus and Colon Health,* Cardiff, CA: Hygeia Publishing, 1995.

Weil, A., *Spontaneous Healing,* New York: Fawcett Columbine, 1995.

Weinreb, E. L., *Anatomy and Physiology,* Reading, MA: Addison Wesley Publishing, 1984.

Weisse, A. B., *The Man's Guide to Good Health,* New York: Consumer Reports Books, 1991.

Weksler, M. E., "Hormone Replacement for Men: Has the Time Come?" *Geriatrics,* 1995: 50 (10): 52–55.

Westheimer, R., *Dr. Ruth's Guide to Good Sex,* New York: Warner Books, 1984.

Weston, L., *Body Rhythm: The Circadian Rhythms Within You,* New York: Harcourt Brace Jovanovich, 1979.

Whitaker, J., *Dr. Whitaker's Guide to Natural Healing:* Rocklin, CA: Prima Publishing, 1995.

Whitecroft, S. I., Crook, D., Marsh, M. S., et al., "Long-Term Effects of Oral and Transdermal Hormone Replacement Therapies on Serum Lipid and Lipoprotein Concentrations," *American Journal of Obstetrics and Gynecology,* 1994, 84:22.

Williams, R., and Williams, V., *Anger Kills,* New York: Random House, 1993.

Williams, R. J., *The Wonderful World Within You,* New York: Bantam Books, 1977.

Winter, A., and Winter, R., *Eat Right, Be Bright,* New York: St. Martin's Press, 1988.

Wright, J., "1994's Secret Health Care Freedom Bill: The Access to Medical Treatment Act," *Let's Live,* Los Angeles, CA, Vol. 62, No. 12, December 1994, p. 70.

Wright, J.V., and Morgenthaler, J., *Natural Hormone Replacement,* Petaluma, CA: Smart Publications, 1997.

Wright, L. S., *Colostrum: Mother Nature's Health Alternative for Every Generation,* Murray, UT: Katchell Publishing, 1998.

Wurtman, J. J., *Managing Your Mind and Mood Through Food,* New York: Rawson Associates, 1986.

Wurtman, J. J., and Suffes, S., *The Serotonin Solution,* New York: Fawcett Columbine, 1996.

Wyatt, G. E., "Child Sexual Abuse and Its Effects on Sexual Functioning," *Annual Review of Sex Research,* 1991: (2): 249–66.

Yedantam, S., "Study Ties Viagra Patients' Heart Ills to Exertion," *Philadelphia Inquirer,* June 1, 2000, p. A22.

Zilbergeld, B., *The New Male Sexuality: The Truth About Men, Sex and Pleasure,* New York: Bantam Books, 1992.

Zonderman, J., and Shader, L., *Nutritional Diseases,* New York: Twenty-First Century Books, 1993.

Zulak, G., "How to Increase Your Muscle Strength, and Manhood—Naturally," *Muscle Mag International,* Hollywood, FL, December 1999, pp. 112–19.

Zussman, L., and Zussman, S., *Getting Together,* New York: William Morrow, 1978.

# Index